OTHER-WORLDLY

MAKING

CHINESE MEDICINE

THROUGH

TRANSNATIONAL

FRAMES

Mei Zhan

Duke University Press   Durham and London   2009

© 2009 Duke University Press

All rights reserved

Printed in the United States of America on acid-free paper ∞

Designed by Heather Hensley

Typeset in Minion Pro by Achorn International

Library of Congress Cataloging-in-Publication data appear
on the last printed page of this book.

An earlier version of chapter 3 appeared in
Cultural Anthropology 16.4 (2001): 453–80.

Duke University Press gratefully acknowledges the support of the
Chiang Ching-Kuo Foundation for International Scholarly Exchange,
which provided funds toward the production of this book.

OTHER-WORLDLY

To my parents
Huang Jingying
and
Zhan Youhua

谁言寸草心
报得三春晖

CONTENTS

PREFACE AND ACKNOWLEDGMENTS

My mother made a big discovery when she was cleaning out the apartment in Shanghai where her late father had lived. Among her father's medical files were three *gaofang* written between 1985 and 1987. Gaofang, or "prescription of rich paste," typically consists of thirty to forty tonifying herbs to be cooked into a thick paste, stored in a sealed jar, and consumed daily for forty to fifty days beginning on the winter solstice. Because of the complexity of gaofang it is prescribed exclusively by experienced herbal doctors. My mother could barely contain her excitement when she asked me over the phone, "Can you guess who wrote these prescriptions for your grandfather? It's someone you know."

I was carried back to the winters of 1998 and 1999, when as part of my translocal and multi-sited field research on traditional Chinese medicine I followed several herbalists as each of them traveled to and practiced at multiple clinics and hospitals in Shanghai. In the weeks leading to the winter solstice, they added extra clinic hours to meet the spike in demand for gaofang, which having long been popular among the elderly was now beginning to attract members of the emerging young urban middle class who found their health compromised by their stressful lives and careers. The name of one practitioner stood out for me, "Is it Dr. He Liren?"[1]

I guessed right. Today—four days after the conversation with my mother—three pieces of pink paper arrived through

A *gaofang* written for the author's grandfather by Dr. He Liren.

international express mail at my home in Irvine, California, where I was finishing my ethnography of the "worlding" of traditional Chinese medicine. I unfolded the first of the three papers. Prescriptions for herbal medicine and acupuncture at clinics and hospitals of traditional Chinese medicine in Shanghai were usually filled out on printed forms that required standardized traditional Chinese diagnostics along with a biomedical diagnosis. This gaofang, in contrast, was entirely handwritten except for the name of the hospital. Read from right to left, up and down, it included a detailed diagnostic narrative of my grandfather's health conditions, a prescription of medicinal herbs and animal products, and even instruction for how to prepare and store the paste. The personal seal of He Liren was stamped at the beginning of the text and another one was stamped at the end. A third seal, which read *jixiang yannian* (good fortune and longer life), was placed in the lower left corner.

As I read the gaofang I could almost visualize Dr. He sitting at his desk in his white lab coat. Surrounded by patients, he would explain to me from time to time how he had reached a particular diagnosis and prescription. Just as important, if not more so, I learned from him things about Chinese medicine well beyond—and yet still intimately entangled with—practices of diagnosis and prescription inside the clinic. He reminisced how in 1959 he and his classmates at the newly founded Shanghai College of Traditional Chinese Medicine labored together to lay down the foundation for the Longhua Hospital of Traditional Chinese Medicine. Forty years later, however, as the academic dean of the Shanghai University of Traditional Chinese Medicine, he was constantly fretting over his own students' apparent indifference toward Chinese medicine. One of our last long conversations took place after Dr. He returned from a visit at the Meridian Institute, a college of traditional Chinese medicine in Monterey, California, founded by an

American cardiovascular surgeon.[2] Though Dr. He was discreet in his comments about acupuncture and herbal medicine in the United States, Dr. He became animated when talking about how inspired he was by the conversational "California-style" pedagogy, which seemed to stimulate students' interest in their studies.

In spite of the many conversations we shared, the fact that Dr. He had treated my grandfather came to me as a surprise and revelation. My acquaintance with Dr. He, or for that matter my inquiry into the shifting discourses, practices, and institutional forms of traditional Chinese medicine, did not have a simple origin story in my family history. In fact, I came to know Dr. He through a very different route that meandered out of the San Francisco Bay Area. In 1995 I met Barbara Bernie, the founding president of the nonprofit American Foundation of Traditional Chinese Medicine, when she gave a guest lecture for a class at Stanford Medical School—a lecture that countered the instructor's aim to debunk "unscientific" and "pseudoscientific" medical practices including Chinese medicine. As my fieldwork in San Francisco unfolded, I began working as a volunteer at the American Foundation of Traditional Chinese Medicine. There I met Huang Lixin, the enterprising president of the American College of Traditional Chinese Medicine in San Francisco and a frequent traveler between China and the United States. Shortly before I left for Shanghai in summer 1998, President Huang wrote a letter that introduced me to a contact of hers in Shanghai—namely, Dr. He Liren.

I was already in the middle before I knew that I had begun. The arrival of Dr. He's gaofang was a moment that saw disparate routes tangled up, unlikely intersections rendered visible, origins relocated and made to multiply, temporalities reshuffled, and an ethnography that was about to close—if it were going to "close" at all—suddenly reopened and plotted anew. This was not a moment outside of—or a world parallel to—my ethnographic account of the worlding of traditional Chinese medicine: a set of translocal, world-making projects and processes of knowledge production deeply embedded in shifting visions and constitutions of the worlds we inhabit. Instead, it was part and parcel of it in ways both unexpected and yet perfectly imaginable. I am certainly not the first anthropologist to have been caught up in serendipitous moments in research and writing. My aim here, however, is to place socialities of both expected and unexpected encounters, entanglements, displacements, and ruptures at the center of this ethnography instead of treating them as unstructured, fortuitous anecdotes and thereby relegating them to the peripheries of ethnographic writing and anthropological imagination.

This book could not have been written without my concerns and fascinations with questions of "traditional Chinese medicine," "knowledge," "China," and "globalization." Yet my work is not so much an exercise in developing a theory of any of these topics as it is committed to exploring ways of reimagining ethnographic possibilities and reformulating anthropological questions, in particular a translocal analytic that allows us to coimagine, rather than enclose, and to anticipate, rather than predict, the always emergent worlds of knowledge with all of their contradictions and contingencies. Without attempting to reunite and articulate simultaneously questions of both ontological and epistemological natures, my work in this volume simply tries to see how we would get on without starting from this divide in the first place. Knowledge making—including the making of anthropological and medical knowledges—is world making. And I could not have asked for a more fitting ending/beginning of this ethnography of knowledge production than the arrival of Dr. He's gaofang.

This book, together with those who have shaped its making, is part of the worlding of traditional Chinese medicine. In Sylvia Yanagisako and Lisa Rofel I found the kind of mentors and friends of whom any fledgling intellectual would dream. Since its conceptualization, they inspired and pushed this project forward in ways most exciting and challenging to me, and sustained it with sound advice. Dan Segal taught me the first things I knew about anthropology, nurtured me along the way, and urged me to keep an eye out for the unexpected in both fieldwork and analysis. David Sadava brought me into his biology lab to study Chinese herbs, thereby sending me on my way to pursue anthropological studies of science and medicine. I am grateful to Linda Barnes, Charlotte Furth, Dorinne Kondo, and Hugh Raffles for their warm encouragement, exhaustive and meticulous comments, fine eye for ethnographic details, and creative and critical insights—at least some of which, I hope, are reflected in this ethnography. Ann Anagnost, Don Brenneis, Tim Choy, Lawrence Cohen, Monica De-Hart, Judith Farquhar, Elisabeth Hsu, Stacey Langwick, Ralph Litzinger, and Volker Scheid have all been invaluable interlocutors who sharpened my thinking and nudged this project in fresh directions. I am also indebted to the three anonymous reviewers whose constructive criticism, illuminating comments, and generous encouragement have helped mold the book into its final form. Ken Wissoker's enthusiasm, support, and thoughtful and thought-provoking input made the writing process a thoroughly enjoyable and rewarding experience for me.

I could not have written this book without the support of my wonderful colleagues at the University of California, Irvine. Victoria Bernal, Tom Boellstorff, Susan Greenhalgh, and Bill Maurer initiated and organized writing groups—mostly for my benefit I suspect—where they pushed this book along with gentle critiques, inspired suggestions, and good humor. Teresa Caldeira, Leo Chavez, Susan Coutin, Lara Deeb, Jim Ferguson, Inderpal Grewal, Karen Leonard, Liisa Malkki, George Marcus, Michael Montoya, Kavita Phillip, Ken Pomeranz, Dorothy Solinger, Kaushik Sunder Rajan, Jenny Terry, Wang Feng, and Jeff Wasserstrom were generous with their comments and encouragements. At Stanford University, Jane Collier and Matthew Kohrman read, critiqued, and helped reshape many of the earlier drafts that became this book. George Collier, Lynn Eden, Joan Fujimura, Akhil Gupta, Miyako Inoue, and Purnima Mankekar helped me conceptualize and reexamine my research and writing. Many conversations and excellent dinners with Monica DeHart, Arzoo Osanloo, Anu Sharma, and Scott Wilson over the years compelled me to keep on writing—and imagining—especially when it seemed difficult. Throughout all this, Ellen Christensen made me feel at home.

This book would not exist without the practitioners of traditional Chinese medicine in both Shanghai and the San Francisco Bay Area who generously shared with me their time and knowledge, hopes and fears. I was most fortunate to be their student, interlocutor, and friend. Throughout this book pseudonyms are given to them to protect their identities, with the exception of those who are readily recognizable public figures. Whereas I cannot fully express my gratitude to each and every one of them in the text of the book, I would like to thank, in particular, Bao Zhijun, Gu Naiqiang, He Liren, He Yumin, Ma Zhongjie, Pang Panchi, Ruan Wangchun, Tong Yao, Wang Shihui, and Wu Hongzhou at the hospitals and medical universities in Shanghai; Huang Lixin and Cheryl Sterling at the American College of Traditional Chinese Medicine; the late Barbara Bernie at the American Foundation of Traditional Chinese Medicine; and DaRen Chen,

John Kao, Laurel Kao, Lam Kong, Howard Kong, Situ Hansun, Min Ting, and Lloyd Wright, who helped me with my research in the San Francisco Bay Area.

My fieldwork for this project was funded by the National Science Foundation Science and Technology Studies Program, the Social Science Research Council International Field Dissertation Research Fellowship, the Wenner-Gren Foundation for Anthropological Research Predoctoral Grant, and the Department of Cultural and Social Anthropology at Stanford University. In addition, various stages of the writing process were funded by the Mac-Arthur Consortium Fellowship in International Peace and Cooperation and the Mellon Dissertation Fellowship, both administered through Stanford University, as well as a Faculty Career Development Award from the University of California.

Pascal Gimenez saw me through the completion of this book with a big heart and many home-made chocolate soufflés. My parents, Huang Jingying and Zhan Youhua, are largely responsible for how I turned out and who I am today. I dedicate this book—a most insignificant tribute—to my parents whose unyielding love, understanding, and support have sustained me all through my life and whose meaning to me is simply beyond the power of words.

INTRODUCTION

This book is an ethnography of translocal knowledge production. In it I write about how dynamic forms of traditional Chinese medicine emerge through particular kinds of encounters and entanglements, which also produce uneven visions, understandings, and practices of what makes up the world and our places in it. Conventional depictions of traditional Chinese medicine have often assumed it to be an enduring system of therapeutic knowledge marked by unique attributes, a system which in recent years has been swept up by globalization. I highlight this point instead: what we have come to call "traditional Chinese medicine" is made *through*—rather than prior to—various translocal encounters and from discrepant locations.[1]

When acupuncture needles enter the skin and when herbal soups are ingested, they do more than adjust the flow of *qi*, generate endorphins, or release a variety of active pharmaceutical ingredients; they also conjure specific and powerful imaginaries of our worlds. An anthropological inquiry into the shifting discourses and practices of Chinese medicine requires venturing into meaningful projects of mapping, temporalizing, and positioning that produce irreducibly complex and contingent everyday socialities that traverse and exceed the confines of "knowledge" as a contained or containable epistemological domain. This ethnography is thus translocal and multi-sited, not only because it comes out of my fieldwork both inside and outside of clinics and schools of traditional Chinese medicine in Shanghai and the San Francisco Bay Area but also, and more importantly, in its focus on the processes of entwinement, rupture, and displacement in the formation and deployment of knowledges, identities, and communities. Inserted at the intersection of discussions of globalization, knowledge production, and politics of difference, my work in this book strives to coimagine rather than transcend the entangled worlds of traditional Chinese medicine.

Encounters and Entanglements

In July 1971 acupuncturists in Beijing, China, inserted their needles into the American journalist James Reston to relieve postsurgical pain after his emergency appendectomy. From his bed in the Anti-Imperialist Hospital, founded as Peking Union Medical College Hospital by the Rockefeller Foundation in 1921 and renamed in 1966 at the onset of the Cultural Revolution,[2] Reston reported on his extraordinary encounter with traditional Chinese medicine in a front-page article in the *New York Times*:

> I was in considerable discomfort if not pain during the second night after the operation, and Li Chang-yuan, doctor of acupuncture at the hospital, with my approval, inserted three long thin needles into the outer part of my right elbow and below my knees and manipulated them in order to stimulate the intestine and relieve the pressure and distension of the stomach. That sent ripples of pain racing through my limbs and, at least, had the effect of diverting my attention from the distress in my stomach. Meanwhile, Doctor Li lit two pieces of an herb called ai, which looked like the burning stumps of a broken cheap cigar, and held them close to my abdomen while occasionally twirling the needles into action. All this took about 20 minutes, during which I remember thinking that it was a rather complicated way to get rid of gas in the stomach, but there was noticeable relaxation of the pressure and distension within an hour and no recurrence of the problem thereafter. (1971:1)

Reston's trip to China was followed by Richard Nixon's historic visit seven months later, and by American scientists and biomedical practitioners who became intrigued by his report that herbal medicine and especially acupuncture not only were used for pain relief, arthritis, and paralysis, but also were cures for deafness and blindness.[3] On their arrival, many of these first-time visitors were captivated by clinical demonstrations such as acupuncture anesthesia—a newly invented procedure in which acupuncture and moxibustion (the burning of the herb *ai*, or mugwort leaf) were used in place of chemical anesthetics during surgery.

Sensational as it might have been, acupuncture was not the only thing that impressed the American visitors, who realized that, contrary to their expectations, they did not land in a communist China hidden behind the bamboo curtain and isolated from the rest of the world. As Reston himself was quick to note, "Despite its name and all the bitter political slogans on the walls, the [Anti-Imperialist] Hospital is an intensely human and vibrant institution. It is not exactly what the Rockefeller Foundation had in mind when it created the Peking Union Medical College, but like everything else in China these days, it is on its way toward some different combination of the very old and the very new" (6).

Reston was not alone in his observation of the vibrant activities at hospitals in China. When I began my preliminary fieldwork on Chinese medicine in the San Francisco Bay Area in 1995, I met many acupuncturists and biomedical professionals who visited hospitals—especially hospitals of traditional Chinese medicine—in China in the years leading to and immediately following the normalization of Sino-U.S. relations in 1979. Having prepared themselves for an encounter with an ancient culture, an isolated communist state, and an exotic healing practice, they were instead overwhelmed by the ubiquitous presence of students, medical professionals, and other travelers from Africa, Southeast Asia, and Latin America. Some of these Third World sojourners were on short visits, whereas others were undergoing formal training in acupuncture. As my interviewees from the Bay Area told me: "There was a world there, although of an unfamiliar kind!"

Fascinated by these stories of other-worldly encounters, I was quickly pulled into the networks and routes from which they emerged. When I first started designing an ethnographic project on the current transformations of traditional Chinese medicine, I had a single field site in mind. I thought that the San Francisco Bay Area would be ideal, where the popularity of acupuncture and herbal medicine—along with other forms of "complementary and alternative medicine" (CAM)[4]—was surging through patient demands, sustained and new laboratory and clinical research, expansion in educational and clinical institutions, legislative support, and increasingly embrasive health insurance coverage. However, when I talked to practitioners and students of traditional Chinese medicine in the Bay Area it was clear that many traveled back and forth across the Pacific and many others aspired to do so. Experiences of China, whether real, imagined, or anticipated, were part and parcel of their everyday practice. By the time I set off for Shanghai in 1998, my project had become decidedly translocal and multi-sited as I moved back and forth between Shanghai and San Francisco and between various hospitals, clinics, colleges, and many more unexpected places. Most important, I was deeply enmeshed in the ever-shifting worlds of traditional Chinese medicine.

Once in Shanghai, I found myself surrounded by a dizzying array of action. Shuguang Hospital, one of the three regular teaching hospitals of the Shanghai University of Traditional Chinese Medicine (SUTCM), was one of the lively places where I conducted much of my participant observation.[5] It was established in 1954, two years before the founding of the university itself. In the 1970s and 1980s it was a hub for foreign visitors and, with the support of the World Health Organization (WHO) and the Chinese Ministry of Health, it provided systematic acupuncture training to international students, especially those from developing countries in Africa, Latin America, and Southeast Asia. By the end of the 1990s, however, Shuguang Hospital had become part of a burgeoning world of a startlingly different contour. It was sandwiched on one side by the bustling, ultratrendy Huai-hai Road where one glistening skyscraper after another came to dominate the landscape; on the other side it was flanked by rows of crumbling two-story residential buildings in the process of being torn down to make way for more modern things.[6]

This was a familiar sight when I looked out of the windows of the Department of Acupuncture (*zhenjiuke*) and the Department of General Internal Medicine (*puneike*), the latter of which specializes in the herbal treatment of a wide array of internal illness ranging from the common cold to cancer. Both departments were on the fourth floor of the clinic building. Whereas General Internal Medicine was often overwhelmed with patients—many of whom were from the disappearing neighborhood below—the Department of Acupuncture was preoccupied with receiving foreign visitors and with training throngs of overseas students, especially those on short-term acupuncture programs.[7] Unlike their Third World predecessors of the 1970s and 1980s, these foreign students were mostly from North America, Europe, Japan, and Korea. To accommodate these newcomers, Shuguang Hospital gave the Department of Acupuncture a special locker room and lounge complete with leather couches, which became something of an envy among the herbalists who had to change their clothes behind a screen in the back of the treatment room. The herbal doctors resigned to the tongue-in-cheek rhetoric that having a nice lounge was a matter of "national honor" with so many foreign students and visitors from "developed and affluent countries" (*fada guojia*) coming and going all the time.

In spite of the enthusiasm from foreign visitors and students, as well as the institutions and organizations that helped set up international acupuncture programs, not everyone agreed that acupuncture was the undisputable essence and pride of traditional Chinese medicine. While I was working at the Department of Acupuncture I often saw confused patients asking the nurses, "Where can I find 'Chinese medicine' (*zhongyi*)?" Without hesitation, the nurses would point their fingers away from the Department of Acupuncture and toward Internal Medicine at the other end of the hallway. The nurses' gestures all but gave away their own assumption, at those particular moments of interaction at least, that herbal medicine rather than acupuncture stood for Chinese medicine. This opinion seemed well supported by the patients who had been turned away: none of them came back. However, the nurses did not always stick to the same interpretation and deployment of what counts as Chinese medicine: when acupuncture patients asked why there were so many foreigners in the treatment room and why they should trust these foreigners to stick needles into their bodies, the nurses would assure them that the foreigners came all the way to the hospital to learn and practice authentic zhongyi and that their presence was merely part of the everyday routine. The essence of Chinese medicine was as elusive and beguiling as the unfamiliar worlds that unfolded before the eyes of James Reston and other American visitors.

These stories bring into focus the unexpected encounters, dislocated actors, entangled knowledges, situated dialogues, and fragile networks that make up traditional Chinese medicine. As I followed practitioners, patients, research scientists, healthcare activists, and bureaucrats across various institutions and networks in Shanghai and the San Francisco Bay Area, "traditional Chinese medicine" worked less and less adequately as the definition for the complex lives and practices that refused to be enclosed within or compartmentalized by any system of knowledge. The words "traditional," "Chinese," and "medicine" are themselves sources of complexity and contingency, especially in the ways in which they are assembled and deployed in everyday discourse and practice. These terms are not self-evident explanations, but rather provisional outcomes of specific kinds of encounters and entanglements that need to be critically analyzed. My aim in this ethnography is not to provide a social history of traditional Chinese medicine: the idea of a "social" history already assumes the boundary and interiority of a relatively stable, enduring core of knowledge and its exteriority.[8] Neither do I intend to dwell exclusively on clinics and medical texts as privileged sites of knowledge production. Instead I strive for broader and more fluid conceptions and analyses of knowledge making by focusing on translocal projects and processes that traverse ethnographic and analytical scales.

To do so, I draw on a wide range of cultural theories, especially theories and methodologies developed in feminist anthropology and in anthropological studies of science, which have been particularly good at crossing forbidding boundaries and laying bare otherwise unapparent connections and ruptures. Specifically, I think of feminist and anthropological studies of science as a mode of analysis and a line of inquiry rather than a discipline bounded by (arti)facts and practices that can readily lay claim to the status of technoscience. "Science Studies" is invoked here as a way of asking different questions about traditional Chinese medicine. Instead of privileging new technologies or new historical milieus as obvious sources of—or explanations for—transformation and novelty, I am interested in the creative and meaningful ways in which shifting networks and forms of traditional Chinese medicine are assembled and reassembled, and how these networks can sometimes take the translocal trajectories of traditional Chinese medicine—and my account of it—into unexpected directions.

My expansive conception of knowledge and my analytical orientation toward relations and processes has also enabled me to write against what I call "reductive globalism"—the prevailing idea that "globalization" is an irreversible process grounded in late-capitalist global economic restructuring, and that the "global" is an all-encompassing spatiotemporal system attainable by ethnographic investigation only indirectly through the studies of the local and the particular. What happens when we refrain from taking the global for granted as a ubiquitous spatiotemporal context within which knowledge production takes place, or as a stable frame of reference for investigations into translocality? Ethnography, I think, can and should have a say about the global itself—or rather, competing visions, understandings, and makings of the global. Is it possible, I ask, not to think about the global as a spatiotemporal inevitability but as emergent socialities entangled in dynamic imaginaries of pasts, futures, and presents? What might be the specific ways in which multiple worlds are envisioned, constituted, and experienced in everyday life on the ground? How can we talk about knowledge production and identity politics without privileging "local culture" as the location of specificities and differences? How can we speak of the global without resorting to narratives of transition and transcendence? How can we take seriously the persisting discourses of East and West, tradition and modernity, culture and science, past and future, and local and global without letting these tropes constrain and cripple our own ethnographic analyses?

In thinking through these questions, I offer an ethnographic account of the translocal movements, displacements, and refigurations—or what I call "worlding"—of traditional Chinese medicine: an exploration of specific world-making projects as emergent, transformative relations and processes deeply and inexorably enmeshed in sociohistorically contingent productions of difference. The worlding of traditional Chinese medicine is not about how a local system of therapeutic knowledge expands into other corners of the world by transcending geopolitical limits and cultural boundaries. The routes of Chinese medicine resemble nothing like a seamless circuit; rather, they take many unexpected turns, burst at the seams, and carve out new landscapes while recharting old ones.

Translocality

This volume comes out of a decade of fieldwork in Shanghai and the San Francisco Bay Area. Beginning in 1995, and most intensively from July 1998 to December 1999, I conducted field research among communities of traditional Chinese medicine. In Shanghai, I carried out most of my institutionally based participant observation at SUTCM and Shuguang Hospital. In the city of San Francisco, I worked mainly at two institutions: the American Foundation of Traditional Chinese Medicine (AFTCM), a nonprofit organization that played leading roles in the education, dissemination, and legislation of traditional Chinese medicine and that provided consultation services to biomedical hospitals; and the American College of Traditional Chinese Medicine (ACTCM), the only college of traditional Chinese medicine in San Francisco. I worked intermittently as a volunteer at AFTCM from 1996 to 2002, audited classes at SUTCM, and worked and studied as an "intern" at Shuguang Hospital and the ACTCM community clinic between 1998 and 1999.[9]

At the same time that I worked with these institutions I followed practitioners and advocates who traveled through and across various institutional and social networks to practice, teach, and promote Chinese medicine. In both Shanghai and the Bay Area, well-established practitioners tend also to be frequent travelers: practicing and teaching at multiple clinics and hospitals (including units within biomedical hospitals such as pain management centers or departments of Chinese medicine); networking with government agencies, commercial interests, and NGOs; engaging in community outreach activities; presenting work at professional forums; and going abroad—including flying across the Pacific—for conferences and workshops.[10] It is no exaggeration to say that extensive traveling mediates as well as measures the success of practitioners.

Like the practitioners of traditional Chinese medicine, I try to think through rather than between or within Shanghai and San Francisco.[11] My work in this ethnography is translocal without taking translocality to be an intermediate scale of circulation conveniently nestled between the local and the global. "Translocal" is not the same as "trans-locale" and "trans-national," which are suggestive of an ontological and analytical priority of places and practices of "dwelling" (Clifford 1992) over place-making projects and processes.[12] This account of translocality builds on the emergent body of ethnographies that calls attention to transnational cultural processes, routes, and uneven fields of power often neglected by discussions of globalization (Ho 2006; Kondo 1997; Piot 1999; Lionnet and Shih 2005; Rofel 2007; Tsing 2005), that remind us of forgotten, marginalized and nonetheless compelling imaginaries of the world (Ferguson 2006; Karl 2002), and that develop the translocal as an analytical position and strategy (Boellstorff 2005; Bowen 2004; Gupta and Ferguson 1992, 1997; Grewal 2005).

Moreover, my emphasis on translocality takes seriously seemingly serendipitous moments and turns in the everyday practice of Chinese medicine. As such, this ethnography is oriented toward encounters and entanglements that are as much about incongruence and disjuncture as they are about movement and connection of both anticipated and unanticipated sorts. As the practitioners, students, and advocates of Chinese medicine led me to predictable institutional sites such as colleges and clinics, I found myself constantly caught up in moments of disjuncture or surprising connections: health fairs at high-tech corporations in Silicon Valley where acupuncturists showcased their trade alongside chiropractors and healthcare insurance companies (chapter 1); medical scandals and contentious relations among practitioners as well as with their patients (chapter 2); clinical "miracles" that defy death sentences made by biomedical professionals (chapter 3); creative translational practices through which new forms of knowledges and authorities emerge (chapter 4); daughters of families of traditional Chinese medicine who creatively negotiated gender and kinship relations and in so doing professional identities (chapter 5); and international conferences that divided as much as they brought together practitioners and advocates from diverse locations (chapter 6). Unexpected encounters are not merely anomalies or exceptions in the structure of Chinese medicine, but rather are constitutive of the very fabric of its worlds by rendering these worlds irreducibly complex and perpetually open-ended. To coimagine the worlds of Chinese medicine, as well as the works and lives of those who produce and inhabit them, necessitates an analytic that embraces these dense moments of encounters including the ruptures and surprises that come along with them. After all, what is life without its effervescent moments?

Unbinding "Traditional Chinese Medicine"

Among the first Americans who visited SUTCM were a group of U.S.-trained acupuncturists from San Francisco. Their trip was arranged by what later became AFTCM. Barbara Bernie, the founding president, herself led the group on their first trip. I first met Barbara in 1996 when she gave a guest lecture at a class on CAM at Stanford University—a class that was taught by a retired surgeon. Even though most of the students in the class, myself included, expected to learn about alternative therapeutic practices, we were in for a surprise when the curriculum did little else than, in the instructor's words, make an effort at "debunking unscientific and pseudoscientific medical systems and claims," including traditional Chinese medicine. It turned out that the instructor, who had been to Shanghai several times, was actively involved in organizations and publications that dismissed traditional Chinese medicine as a politically motivated invention by the Chinese communist government and, ironically, as a fraud because it contained too many biomedical elements.

Barbara arrived armed with illustrations of the meridian system and the five-element chart, and she stood her ground as the instructor pestered her with questions and attempted to discredit both her and Chinese medicine as a whole. In the end the class applauded her and so did I. Soon afterward, I began volunteering at AFTCM and came to know Barbara well over the next six years. She grew up in an upper-middle-class Russian Jewish immigrant family in New York, but then moved to San Francisco at the end of the 1960s with her husband, who ran a successful manufacturing business. On her arrival she insisted on interviewing potential candidates before selecting a family physician. In thinking of this decision she noted, "What I did was quite unusual back then. Some of the physicians simply hung up on me!"

In 1970 Barbara came down with a mysterious illness. She was tired all of the time, could not concentrate, and had a constant headache. Her physicians could not determine what was ailing her, even after running many laboratory tests. Although her ailment most likely was chronic fatigue syndrome, it was not until 1988 that the term entered biomedical vocabulary and became an identifiable disease often associated with urban middle-class lifestyles.[13] After her physicians told her that there was little to do to help, she went to Vancouver B.C. on a friend's advice and was cured by an acupuncturist who had immigrated there from Singapore. Decades later she would continue to say, "What a wonderful medicine! I was determined that everybody in the United States should know about it, and whoever wants it should be able to have it."

After recovering from her illness, Barbara pursued training in acupuncture first in Britain, where she was influenced by Jack Worsley's Five Element Acupuncture (see chapter 1), and then in the Bay Area, where she worked with the acupuncturist Miriam Lee, a Chinese immigrant from Singapore. She participated in the grassroots movement to legalize acupuncture by giving lectures on the radio, for example, and by testifying in Sacramento after Lee was arrested in 1974 for practicing without a license.[14] After acupuncture was legalized in the state of California in 1975, Barbara became one of the first licensed acupuncturists. In reflecting on her first trip to China in 1977, Barbara stated: "I had gone looking for authentic Chinese medicine. I was so excited and all I wanted was to learn." She was shocked, however, to find out that her hosts—who were university professors well trained in natural science—were highly skeptical of acupuncture. She told me, "I ended up in my hotel room educating my Chinese friends about the virtues of acupuncture. I bought some acupuncture needles, and even started treating some of the Chinese people who came to see me!"

The question of authenticity and change has long been at the heart of the debates over how to understand traditional Chinese medicine. Although recent popular discourses in both China and the United States often present traditional Chinese medicine as an ancient therapeutic healing system and practice that first emerged in China "thousands of years" ago, others—especially opponents of traditional Chinese medicine in the United States—accuse it of being nothing more than a politically motivated invention by the Chinese Communist Party. Within academia, the double bind of antiquity and novelty has also troubled historical and anthropological inquiries into the transformations of traditional Chinese medicine. The historian Paul Unschuld, for example, argues that traditional Chinese medicine consists of a "durable paradigmatic core" and a "soft coating of therapeutic knowledge" that adapts to different social and historical conditions (1985: 7–8). This core-and-coating model helps incorporate "change" into the analysis of traditional Chinese medicine, even if it does so by maintaining the separation between knowledge and practice, text and context, and the primordial and the hybrid.

In recent years, analytical focus has shifted toward a more direct engagement with the heterogeneity and historicity of the knowledges of traditional Chinese medicine (e.g., Andrews 1996; Barnes 1995, 2005; Farquhar 1987, 1994; Hsu 1999; Lei 1999; Scheid 2002, 2007; Taylor 2005). This body of scholarship emphasizes that traditional Chinese medicine cannot be reduced to a self-contained, coherent system that is then presumed to be emblematic of an ancient Chinese culture. Nor is Chinese medicine the antithesis or prototype of modern Western science. Instead, this literature investigates how traditional Chinese medicine is positioned vis-à-vis discourses of tradition, modernity, science, and biomedicine. Some examine the institutionalization of traditional Chinese medicine and the nationwide efforts at standardizing it in the form of TCM during and after the communist revolution (Hsu 1999; Taylor 2005). Some highlight the interaction and entanglement between the institutional forms, discourses, and practices of traditional Chinese medicine and Western medicine (Andrews 1996; Barnes 2003; Farquhar 1994; Kaptchuk 2000). Some stress the relation between the development of traditional Chinese medicine and politics of modernity and nationalism (Andrews 1996; Lei 1999). There has also been an increasing interest in the entrepreneurship and commodification of Chinese medicine (Farquhar 1995; Hsu 2002), as well as how Chinese medicine is invented and refigured through modern technologies (Scheid 2002).

All of these discussions have helped situate the practice of traditional Chinese medicine socially and historically, and they draw out the complex politics of difference at stake in the discourses and practices of traditional

Chinese medicine. This ethnography builds on this body of literature by foregrounding Chinese medicine "in action." This means, first, an attentiveness to the everyday worlds of Chinese medicine—those not limited to the clinical and pedagogical but also embracive of contestatory processes of how knowledges, identities, and communities are differently constituted. Second, and more important, it means to rethink Chinese medicine as a set of contingent products of particular kinds of socialities.

Many scholars have noted the influence of biomedicine on traditional Chinese medicine in terms of conceptual framing, institution building, clinical and pedagogical practice, laboratory research, insurance policies, and legislation. In this volume I take the analysis of encounters and entanglements one step further by placing them at the very center of the discourses, practices, and institutions of traditional Chinese medicine. Interactions with biomedical professionals, relations with patients who move back and forth between biomedicine and traditional Chinese medicine, and negotiations with healthcare policies and legislatures are not just occasional incidents but rather are the everydayness of Chinese medicine. It is through these encounters, mundane and extraordinary at the same time, that the very "core" of traditional Chinese medicine takes on specific shapes. This book is set against the background of three such core-forming historical moments.

First, the 1910s and 1920s saw the expansion of biomedical ideologies and institutions in China and, as a response, the emergence of professional organizations and private institutions of traditional Chinese medicine for the first time in history. As Bridie Andrews (1996) notes, however, this expansion was not the consequence of the "multiplication of contexts" of Western science either by westerners or by Chinese people trained to Western standards. Instead it came about as a result of the relevance of biomedicine to the specific and sometimes divergent interests of the Chinese state as well as those of scholars, politicians, and medical professionals. This brand of Western medicine came to be known as "new medicine" (*xinyi*). At the same time, the terms "old medicine" (*jiuyi*) and "national medicine" (*guoyi*) began appearing in both written and spoken languages to lump together a wide range of therapeutic practices—herbal medicine, acupuncture, therapeutic massage (*tuina*), bone setting, and healing rituals among others. Whereas the opponents of Chinese medicine favored the term "jiuyi", the proponents purposefully used guoyi to connote a sense of national essence and pride. These naming practices simultaneously universalized the West and the knowledge production associated with it and invented its objectified, culturally bounded, antiquated Other.

During the first half of the twentieth century, members of the Nationalist Party government launched several campaigns to eliminate jiuyi, which in their view was the obstacle that stood in the way of healthcare reform and modernization (Lei 1999; Qiu 1998). In protest, practitioners in urban areas—especially Shanghai, which since becoming a treaty port at the end of the Opium War in 1843 had been drawing migrants including established healers from nearby provinces—started forming professional organizations and setting up small, private academies of traditional Chinese medicine.[15] Drawing on the administrative, curricular, and pedagogical styles of biomedicine, the herbalist Ding Ganren and others founded the Shanghai Professional School of Traditional Chinese Medicine (Shanghai Zhongyi Zhuanmen Xuexiao) in 1916. In addition, two other small, private academies of traditional Chinese medicine were also founded in Shanghai: the Shanghai College of Traditional Chinese Medicine (Shanghai Zhongguo Yixueyuan) in 1928 and the Shanghai College of New Traditional Chinese Medicine (Shanghai Xinzhongguo Yixueyuan) in 1936. These schools were well regarded—even at the end of the 1990s the schools' surviving alumni, by then in their seventies and eighties, still lovingly called these academies *laosanxiao* ("the three old schools").[16] In 1946, however, the Ministry of Education ordered laosanxiao to close down; according to the government inspectors, the schools suffered from "inadequate equipment and inappropriate management." Students and faculty protested in response, and they continued to hold classes until 1948 (Qiu 1998).

The second wave of institutionalization began in the 1950s. After the founding of the People's Republic of China in 1949, small institutions such as laosanxiao were remembered and mobilized as the foundation of the new state-run colleges and hospitals of traditional Chinese medicine. Many of the graduates of laosanxiao played instrumental roles as administrators, educators, and clinicians—often at the same time—in the founding of the Shanghai College of Traditional Chinese Medicine (SCTCM), one of the first four state-run, large-scale colleges of traditional Chinese medicine in 1956. Today, both official history and senior practitioners in Shanghai recognize laosanxiao as the immediate predecessors of SCTCM, which was renamed SUTCM in 1993.

Significantly, the institutionalization of the 1950s was made possible by adopting the standards and institutional forms of biomedicine. In 1954 Shanghai No. 11 Hospital, a biomedical hospital, became Shuguang Hospital of Traditional Chinese Medicine, thus establishing the first hospital of Chinese medicine. By order of the party-state, biomedical doctors were organized into study groups to learn traditional Chinese medicine from senior herbal doctors and acupuncturists. These biomedical professionals then went on to serve two main functions: first, to run hospitals of traditional Chinese medicine, as most practitioners of traditional Chinese medicine had no experience in this area; and second, to develop a body of scientifically verifiable medical theory for traditional Chinese medicine. In Shanghai, some of these biomedical professionals later reversed back to practicing biomedicine, some began conducting laboratory and clinical research on traditional Chinese medicine, and yet others decided to make traditional Chinese medicine their permanent profession. Indeed, some of today's "old famous doctors of traditional Chinese medicine" (*minglao zhongyi*), officially recognized by the municipality, were from this generation of biomedical professionals.[17] In the 1960s and 1970s this standardized and scientized traditional Chinese medicine, in particular acupuncture, was also exported to Third World countries as part of a low-tech and low-cost preventive medicine for the common people, especially the rural poor. This mass export was mediated by and in turn contributed to China's effort to champion "the proletariat world."

This proletariat world, however, was eclipsed in the third moment of dense translocal encounters, which began in the 1980s. The 1980s saw the shift of the proliferation of traditional Chinese medical practices and institutions away from Third World countries to refocus on Euro-Asian and trans-Pacific routes. At the same time, Chinese medicine was also going through a profound remaking that bifurcated its area of expertise. On the one hand, it had come increasingly to occupy the treatment of illnesses where biomedicine is less effective or ineffective (see chapter 3). On the other hand, Chinese medicine had been reinvented as a new kind of preventive medicine for a new world: no longer targeting the rural poor of the proletariat world of the 1960s and 1970s, this new preventive medicine became intimately associated with the translocal production of hip, middle-class, cosmopolitan lifestyles that emphasize overall well-being and mind-body health (see chapter 1). California has come to the fore in these new health practices and imaginaries of the world, as the professionalization of

Chinese medicine continues to be shaped by politics of identification and relations with the changing biomedical mainstream.[18]

These moments of encounters defy binary narratives of tradition and modernity, East and West, culture and science, and particular and universal. Moreover, compared to environmental discourses that thrive on provisional claims to universals, as Anna Tsing (2005:8) has discussed in her inspiring critique of globalism, the worlding of traditional Chinese medicine takes place through troubled relations (even if not always at odds) with universalistic discourses of biomedicine and science. The claim to universality, which buttresses the production of bioscientific and biomedical authority, has never been a rallying point for Chinese medicine but instead is an ongoing problem: popular and medical discourses often present clinical efficacy and success in Chinese medicine as exceptional cases of "miracles," even as these miracles help traditional Chinese medicine struggle for a space in biomedicine-centered healthcare systems in China and the United States (see chapter 3).

The production of science, then, is not outside of the making of traditional Chinese medicine but rather very much an integral part of it. The entanglements of traditional Chinese medicine, science, and biomedicine call for a cultural analysis that problematizes the division between "science" and "Other" knowledges. Specifically, it asks for reflections on the question of science in anthropology—how anthropological and broader sociohistorical discourses have explored and represented the relations between knowledge, identity, and community, and how in doing so these discourses have crafted "science" and its Others.

The "Third Divide"

As I try to capture the ways in which Chinese medicine is worlded, it has become critical to bring into the conversation insights from both medical anthropology and cultural and social studies of science. Medical anthropology, professionalized in the United States in the 1950s as a subfield of anthropology, was traditionally defined through the studies of non-Western and nonbiomedical conceptions and practices of body, illness, and healing, as well as of healthcare behaviors and practices among ethnic minorities in the United States or non-Western people. Cultural and social studies of science, in contrast, is a relatively young and interdisciplinary field that draws on insights from various disciplines such as history, philosophy, sociology, anthropology, feminist studies, and natural sciences. The field asks questions about the social, cultural, and political enmeshment of science and technology, and in doing so it challenges the boundaries between society and science, culture and nature.

Anthropology is admittedly a late comer in the field of science studies, especially when compared to philosophy, sociology, and history (Franklin 1995; Martin 1994b). Even so, it has left indelible marks on the field by introducing ethnographic accounts that demystify how scientists work and how scientific knowledge and (arti)facts are actually produced (see, e.g., Haraway 1989; Latour and Woolgar 1979; Traweek 1988), and by bringing in cultural analyses of the "culture of no culture" of science (Traweek 1988). It bears mentioning, however, that anthropology's contribution to science studies cannot be reduced to simply lending the tool of ethnography and transplanting the concept of culture. Institutionalized as the "science of man" toward the end of the nineteenth century, anthropology at its inception made the non-Western, non-white, and "primitive" Others its specific subject that in turn helped position it at the lower end of Euro-American academic hierarchies. Anthropology became the marginal and potentially subversive Other within the humanities and social sciences—in terms of both its subject matter and its mode of inquiry—which, especially in the Boasian tradition that laid the foundation for interpretive anthropology, has always had an anti-positivist leaning. The anthropology of science emerged at a time when "studying up" (Nader 1972)—the study of cultures of power rather than those of the powerless, the seemingly familiar rather than the unfamiliar, "here" rather than "there"—came to redefine the scope and mission of anthropology. The call to study up arrived on the tail of anti-colonial, civil rights, and counterculture movements. It involved watchfulness toward the exercise of power in ethnographic research and writing, vigilance when approaching authoritative and normative knowledge claims, eagerness to cross institutional and conceptual barriers limiting the range of subjects and questions of anthropological inquiries, and reflexivity concerning anthropology's own methodological and conceptual entanglements in the knowledge productions and cultural formations it set out to examine. Therefore it is not surprising that, together with feminist studies of science, the anthropology of science tends to emphasize that what we come to know as science is accomplished via sociohistorically contingent processes, and that doing science entails constant negotiation, interaction, and strategic moves.

In keeping with the mission to study up, anthropological studies of science have largely focused on Euro-American discourses, practices, and institutions that readily lay claim to the status of "technoscience"—a term that highlights the inseparability of modern technology and scientific knowledge—although the particular project under investigation might be highly controversial within and beyond scientific communities.[19] In recent years, however, the division of labor between the anthropology of science and medical anthropology is becoming blurred. On the one hand, science studies have begun to examine discourses and practices of technoscience outside of privileged sites in Europe and North America, especially through their engagement with theories of postcoloniality, transnationalism, globalization, and late capitalism.[20] Some of these works have turned their attention to the interface between bioscience, ecology, and indigenous knowledges—in particular, the ways in which categories of universality and local knowledge are renegotiated, contested, and articulated.[21] On the other hand, medical anthropology has ventured out of the comfort zones of relativism and ethnomedicine while holding on to its traditional concerns over difference and diversity, and has come to formulate critical analyses of fundamental assumptions about body, illness, and healing in biomedicine (Good 1994; Kleinman 1995; Lock 1988; Lock and Scheper-Hughes 1987; Young 1982). These groundbreaking works, under the umbrella of "critical medical anthropology," have been taken into various productive directions, with some medical anthropologists becoming increasingly interested in the politics of knowledge production through translocal fields of power and embracing concepts and analytical tools developed by science studies.[22]

My work is aimed at further dislodging the traditional division of labor between medical anthropology and science studies, which I suggest is indicative of what Bruno Latour (1993) calls the "two Great Divides" that have mediated and constrained anthropological inquiries into knowledge production. The first divide is that between nature and culture, society and science; the second divide is that between the modern, Western "Us" who proclaim to have made this divide and the premodern "Them/Others" who do not. Latour argues that these are false divides, for the concept of "modern" itself, designating "a new regime, an acceleration, a rupture, a revolution in time" (10) is premised on the conjoined processes of hybridization and purification. While "hybridization" refers to the proliferation of new types of "hybrids" out of mixing nature and culture, "purification" is the simultaneous denial of the ontological status of the hybrids—a denial that actually provides the condition for their proliferation (10–11).

As Latour takes apart the two Great Divides, his analysis also suggests a third divide—namely, that between the moderns who purify and the Others who do not. For those of us interested in studying knowledge production, several analytical questions arise out of the implication of the third divide. Whereas science studies has been tremendously powerful in bringing nature and culture, science and society, back together and into each other in nuanced and productive ways, how do we talk about knowledge productions in which processes of purification did not happen or are not supposed to have happened? What is the relevance of science studies when confronted with knowledge productions in which nature and culture, knowledge and society are assumed to be deeply entangled and do not need to be reunited through our analyses?

With these questions in mind, in this volume I examine knowledge forms that are always already impure, tenuously modern, and permanently entangled in the networks of people, institutions, histories, and discourses within which they are produced. To do so requires that I bring not just the insights of science studies to bear on medical anthropology, but also that I rethink science studies as a way of posing questions about knowledge forms not readily identifiable as technoscientific. Rather than assuming some inert quality or criterion that makes the "West" the normative conceptual space and referent for science and biomedicine, and thus traditional Chinese medicine the non-Western alternative, it is important to examine the understandings and productions of medical knowledge and science in uneven, interactive, translocal networks and processes that constantly push and disrupt the Great Divides.

Furthermore, how do we ask critical questions about knowledge forms not explicitly marked by conceptual breakthroughs or technological innovations, or knowledge productions where such breakthroughs and innovations are viewed with suspicion as threats to history and authenticity? For example, rather than a triumph or a clear goal to strive after, any innovation—be it acupuncture anesthesia, Chinese formula medicine (*zhongchengyao*),[23] or the reinterpretation of medical theory and philosophy—invariably raises suspicions among practitioners and critics alike over questions of authenticity and thereby validity (He 1990). But are technological and theoretical innovations the only way in which we can imagine the newness of Chinese medicine? Or do we have to fall back on an account of the newness of "social context" and thereby re-create the Great Divides?

I think not. Traditional Chinese medicine is more than what happens inside a clinic, a hospital, a classroom, a textbook, or a laboratory. At the same time, what happens inside a clinic is much larger and sometimes more extraordinary than treating illnesses and passing on clinical know-how. It is essential for a faithful account of the worlding of Chinese medicine to hold onto a critical awareness of the fields of power that have mediated and constrained the worlding of traditional Chinese medicine, and in which multiple strategies of mapping, temporalizing, and positioning take place and always produce something emergent—something "new." Transformative relations are themselves always new.

The Limits of Narratives of Transition and Transcendence

Much of the discussion around the globalization of traditional Chinese medicine has focused, for good reasons, on how Chinese medicine departed from China and traveled to other parts of the world—Africa, Europe, East Asia, and the United States. As I try to sketch the trajectories of Chinese medicine, I find myself continuing to struggle with the out-of-China narrative that seems to haunt the mapping of Chinese medicine. It seems easy, perhaps too easy, to begin the narrative of globalization with a departure from China—the place of origin to be left behind in the globalist narratives of transition and transcendence.

The worlding of traditional Chinese medicine tells a different story of mapping, temporalizing, and locating. In summer 2003 SUTCM relocated its campus across the city from Xuhui District to Pudong District. Xuhui is an older district that is located in the southwest corner of Shanghai, part of which belongs to the original French Concession (1849–1943). Pudong, in contrast, was a largely suburban and agricultural area until it was designated a special economic development zone in 1992. Since that time it has come to symbolize the new Shanghai with its skyscrapers and concentration of financial institutions and high-tech companies funded by overseas capital. The SUTCM campus did not just move to any random part of Pudong; rather, it entered "Medicine Valley" (in reference to Silicon Valley) of the Zhangjiang High-Tech Park, one of the two government-sanctioned high-tech areas in China. Medicine Valley boasts a concentration of biotechnological and pharmaceutical firms, which include both Chinese and foreign ventures.[24]

Whereas the university administrators had the immediate future of their school in mind when they made the move, the broader futuristic outlook of traditional Chinese medicine goes beyond the relocation and reorientation of the SUTCM campus and is echoed by many practitioners and advocates, especially those in the Bay Area. Since the legalization of acupuncture in California in 1975, acupuncture and Chinese herbal medicine have been increasing in popularity and gaining a foothold in the medical mainstream through grassroots movements. Since the mid-1990s in particular, acupuncture has been steadily picked up by medical insurance companies, biomedical hospitals, and medical schools. Many of my interlocutors in the San Francisco Bay Area, including a growing number of biomedical professionals and scientists, share the belief that acupuncture and herbal medicine—as well as other CAM practices—are the future of medicine. I spoke with one retired surgeon who was in the process of setting up a new academy of Chinese medicine in the Bay Area. During our interview, which took place on the flight from San Francisco to Shanghai, he voiced his vision of another kind of "medicine valley": "California has a tradition of being future-oriented. Futurists like you and me believe in multiple ways of knowing. In the postmodern world, things are not simply black and white, right or wrong. Western medicine and Chinese medicine can enhance each other and should join hands."[25]

The optimism of these futuristic discourses, however, belies a deep-seated concern and even anxiety over the current state of traditional Chinese medicine—a view that is painfully felt, especially in China. In stark contrast to the celebratory mood of the relocation of SUTCM, the Chinese State Bureau of Traditional Chinese Medicine announced in January 2006 their application for a World Heritage status from UNESCO.[26] This prompted a nationwide outcry: Is Chinese Medicine, the pride of Chinese culture, near extinction? If so, do we really need to announce this to the world? An official at the State Administration of Traditional Chinese Medicine told me that the majority of the foreign students who went to study "natural science" in China pursued education in traditional Chinese medicine. Why, then, does Chinese medicine blossom elsewhere, especially in North America and Europe, but seem to be dying at home?

The debate over the World Heritage designation, in particular, grew into "China's medicine war" (Magnier 2007). Since 2006, traditional Chinese medicine has come under fierce attack from Zhang Gongyao, a scholar who claimed that he studied Chinese medicine for over thirty years.

Supported by several members of the Chinese Academy of Science, he started an online petition to eliminate traditional Chinese medicine, which he claimed to be "unscientific." The petition ignited an ongoing nationwide debate among the medical communities as well as the general public. It forced the Chinese Ministry of Health and the State Administration of Traditional Chinese Medicine to openly declare Chinese medicine as China's "scientific legacy" and "cultural heritage," thus adding a note of urgency for traditional Chinese medicine to obtain World Heritage status (Deng 2006; Ministry of Health 2006). Yet these official statements have escalated the debate rather than put an end to it. On the popular Chinese website Sina .com a survey completed by 20,888 individuals suggested that although 74 percent supported Chinese medicine only 43 percent would seek it in times of sickness (Sina.com 2006a). Even among those who claimed to be supportive of Chinese medicine, there was a deafening silence on the question of "science": the salvage of Chinese medicine was so easily framed as a matter of upholding cultural heritage and national pride that the ambiguous scientific status of Chinese medicine seemed best left untouched when it concerned public opinion.

In Shanghai, many young students of Chinese medicine cast doubts over the scientific basis of their own profession (see chapters 3 and 5). Professional debates among practitioners are often characterized by perplexity and frustration (He 1990; Qu 2005). Some senior professionals simply shake their heads in resignation when asked about the "ups and downs" in the fortune of Chinese medicine. A few senior practitioners at the end of their careers and lives even refuse to train any student or pass on their knowledge in protest of what they see as the westernization of Chinese medicine. Even the most adamant supporters of traditional Chinese medicine recall past battles with biomedicine, and thus lament that "traditional Chinese medicine is like a frail old man trying to make his way through wind and rain: each step is precarious and any misstep could be fatal" (*Shengming Shibao* 2006). How can Chinese medicine be at once a "frail old man" and a hopeful futuristic endeavor? Using Hugh Raffles's term, how do we make sense of the "anticipatory nostalgia" of things that have not yet—and may never—come to pass? Must the future of Chinese medicine lie tenuously within various "medicine valleys"?

I write at a moment when many anthropological inquiries and ethnographic writings are framed within or staged against the present and imminent "age of globalization." Theorists of globalization argue that even if the global is now still partial, it is only because it has not yet fully encompassed the lived experiences of individuals or the domain of institutional orders and social formations (Sassen 2000:216). Within this framework, the global, the national, the local, and the personal remain distinctive "spheres," each of which describes a spatiotemporal order with internal differentiation and growing mutual imbrications. However, the spatiotemporal order of globalism may inadvertently reproduce narratives of transition and transcendence that relegate to the background specific kinds of translocal networks and encounters by which meaningful knowledges and identities are produced, while at the same time leaving these networks and encounters relatively intact from critical analyses.

A critical analysis of the timespace of traditional Chinese medicine entails considerations of not only multiple spatiotemporalities but also the ways in which they remain the provincial and sometimes contradictory outcomes of specific translocal connectivities.[27] Here I take seriously Bruno Latour's suggestion to think of spatiotemporalities as the products of particular actor-networks of people, things, discourses, and institutions—each of which instead of being merely a stop or transmitter along the route of traveling may lead to new bifurcations and ruptures or become origins of new translations (1993, 2005). Latour argues that "one is not born traditional; one chooses to become traditional by constant innovation. The idea of an identical repetition of the past and that of a radical rupture with any past are two symmetrical results of a single conception of time" (1993:76). In this light, this ethnography emphasizes mapping rather than maps, temporalizing rather than temporality, and world making rather than globalization. The relocations of traditional Chinese medicine in time and space suggest that we need to look beyond the ready-made spatiotemporal order and hierarchy of globalism in order to analytically engage and reflect on the multiple strategies of mapping, locating, and temporalizing that shape the forms and orientations of Chinese medicine. Far from transitioning to a global era and breaking free of messy sociohistorical entanglements, the worlding of traditional Chinese medicine is suspended in discrepant spaces and times that are themselves contingent products of uneven translocal fields of power.

Toward an Ethnography of Worlding

My choice of the word "worlding" is a conscious effort to gain distance from globalist assumptions of totality, transition, and transcendence. Martin

Heidegger (1996) coined the term "worlding" in his thesis of phenomenology to signal that the world takes place in things—a critical awareness of the enmeshment of thing and world. The discussion of worlding has since been taken in various directions. Gayatri Spivak (1985) in her critique of nineteenth-century British imperialism famously invokes the worlding of the "Third World" to argue that colonized people and places, though seemingly remote and pristine, were already an intimate and integral part of English cultural production. Dipesh Chakrabarty (2000) also draws on Heidegger—albeit with a critical eye on the conceptual presence of the West that permeates social theory including postcolonial critique—to use the idea of worlding to talk about the modernist and rationalist mode of knowledge production that privileges the social scientist's analytical relations to the world over lived ones. Chakrabarty argues that in refusing to recognize the enmeshment of the ethnographer and his or her subject in multiple, emergent relations, the modernist mode of knowledge production "obliterates the plural ways of being human that are contained in the very different orientations of the world" (241). Building on these discussions of worlding, some scholars have recently invoked the notion to formulate analytical alternatives to habitual understandings of world history and dominant theories of globalization in Euro-American academia (Gillman, Greusz, and Wilson 2004; Rofel 2007; Segal 2004; Wilson and Connery 2007). This emergent body of interdisciplinary literature contends that truly reflexive and inclusive accounts of the world cannot simply be achieved through a maneuver of multiplication that adds on geographical locales into a singular global narrative, but rather entail a redeployment of comparability—terms of cultural comparison—by attuning it to shifting spatiotemporal relations that elude the finality of globalism.[28]

My ethnography of worlding is informed by these ruminations. I am especially mindful of Chakrabarty's suggestion that there are other forms of memory, other forms of history, and other forms of worlding that have not been—indeed cannot be—accounted for by globalist narratives of transition, development, and spatiotemporal singularity and finality. The emancipatory potentials of globalization, I suggest, do not rest in the production of a world where cultural practices and subjectivities promise to transcend local, regional, and national boundaries, and even cut across gender, class, racial, and ethnic divisions (Appadurai 1991). I rethink the notion of worlding not as a replacement for globalization but as an intervention that disrupts transitional and transcendental discourses of global capitalism, and as a heuristic device to think through the multiple spatiotemporalities in and of knowledge production—that is, multiple and effervescent worlds in the making.

The notion of worlding is committed to an epistemology and ontology of entanglements. Knowing the world, as Heidegger (1996:61) argues, is a kind of being-in-the-world. And this includes the production of anthropological knowledges about the world. The worlding of knowledge calls for an intellectual commitment and a critical sensibility to our own participation and positioning in worlds in the making. More importantly, the nontranscendental and yet open-ended nature of worlds in the making should serve as a constant reminder that the worlds we inhabit are by no means finite—and neither are social inquiries into these worlds. In this sense, any attempt at an overarching explanation might just seem to be in the constant danger of being out of place and out of time. An analytical alternative would be to engage rather than explain and coimagine rather than constrict or contain. I thus think of worlding as a critical analytic: a mode of knowing and being that requires us to stand ready to step out of the world to which we have grown familiar and comfortable and to hold onto our abilities to imagine, engage, and even make other emergent worlds, no matter how inchoate, unruly, extraordinary, or mundane they may seem. In contrast to globalist accounts of the world, worlding is liberating precisely because its refusal to transcend forces us to critically connect with the shiftiing worlds we inhabit and, in doing so, reimagine ethnographic possibilities.

My account of the worlding of traditional Chinese medicine is an attempt at this kind of analytic. This ethnography shows that the worlding of Chinese medicine is as much about relocating a college campus, getting a foothold in middle-class neighborhoods, redefining preventive medicine, and redrawing kinship charts as it is about writing herbal prescriptions and inserting acupuncture needles into the skin. I group the chapters that follow into three parts: "Entanglements," "Negotiations," and "Dislocations." Each speaks to a different theme of the worlding of traditional Chinese medicine.

Part 1, "Entanglements," includes two chapters that explore world-making projects that exceed globalist narratives. In chapter 1, "Get on Track with the World," I trace the multiple, uneven trajectories and shifting meanings of Chinese medicine as a "preventive medicine," and I examine the discrepant visions and practices of what makes up the "world" that emerges from and underscores these trajectories. From the 1960s to the early 1970s, China sent medical teams to the "Third World," especially Africa. Acupuncture in particular was reinvented and praised as a "preventive medicine" for the rural poor. In these efforts the state vigorously promoted African-Chinese "brotherhood" and the vision of a racialized proletariat world that China strove to champion. Since the 1980s, however, East Asia, Europe, and North America have eclipsed Africa to become privileged sites for China's efforts to "get on track with the world"—and for reinventing traditional Chinese medicine. Acupuncture is now widely marketed in California as a naturalistic "preventive medicine" suited for a middle-class, cosmopolitan "lifestyle" that focuses on overall "well-being." Practitioners in Shanghai have quickly tuned into this trend and now market new herbal concepts and products that target the emerging middle class. They promote Chinese medicine as a new preventive medicine with a "Californian" flair.

In chapter 2, "Hands, Hearts, and Dreams," I focus on the ways in which processes of commodification and encounters with biomedicine reshape and challenge traditional Chinese medicine as a practice of "kind heart and kind skills" (*renxin renshu*) in both predictable and unpredictable ways. Although the approach to illness and healing taken by Chinese medicine is often perceived as more "holistic" and "humanistic" than that of biomedicine, commodification and marketization have complicated how practitioners struggle for legal status, rethink pedagogy and the learning process, and redefine their areas of expertise while struggling to maintain their practices as a "profession of kindness." Instead of creating a global circuit of exchange value, translocal processes of commodification take on divergent forms, bring in new actors, and create new opportunities and battlefields where knowledges, careers, and lives are at stake.

The second part of this book, "Negotiations," focuses on the refiguration of the clinical knowledges and authorities of traditional Chinese medicine as it is worlded. Locating a secure space within the biomedicine-dominated cosmopolitan medicine means that the negotiations for medical legitimacy and authority are central to reinventing traditional Chinese medical knowledge and practice. Although many traditional Chinese medicine practitioners consider the authority of biomedicine to be grounded in science, they ask, on the one hand, whether a "traditional," "Chinese" medical practice needs to be or can be proven to be "rational" and "effective" in scientific terms. On the other hand, they also ask how to conceive of a "science" that would encompass traditional Chinese medicine. In chapters 3 and 4

I explore the multiple, competing ways that knowledges and identities are negotiated through the various kinds of networks in which practitioners of traditional Chinese medicine take part.

In chapter 3, "Does It Take a Miracle?" I explore how practitioners negotiate clinical and scientific authorities in the production of "clinical miracles." When demonstrating the medical legitimacy of traditional Chinese medicine, practitioners often point out that traditional Chinese medicine is effective where biomedicine is ineffective or less effective—for example, chronic illnesses and certain types of cancer—and that Chinese medicine can produce "clinical miracles" to defy "death sentences" by biomedical doctors. Opponents of traditional Chinese medicine, however, argue that such incidents are too anecdotal or absurd to meet scientific norms. Using materials from participant observation and interviews from both Shanghai and San Francisco I examine clinical encounters through which "miracles" are produced, and I study how practitioners strategically invoke and interpret these "miracles" in professional and broader sociohistorical contexts. I suggest that it is precisely through the process of marginalization that the everyday clinical efficacy of traditional Chinese medicine comes to be measured in terms of "miracles." Clinical miracle as a source for medical legitimacy at once marks the marginality of Chinese medicine, and disrupts universalist narratives of rationality.

In chapter 4, "Translating Knowledges," I discuss the translational practices by which translocal knowledges and identities are constructed. I focus my discussion on what exactly is taught and learned in the day-to-day clinical shifts of Dr. Huang Jixian, an acupuncturist who has trained international students since the late 1970s. Huang explains her practice in "traditional" terms when interacting with students because as she and many students argue, "the students are here to learn traditional medicine." Yet, she consistently uses biomedical language when talking to biomedical colleagues visiting from abroad. I pay specific attention to the ways in which knowledges and meanings are produced through these translational practices, and I argue that translation is not a neutral medium that bridges existing cultural differences but rather is a set of uneven, contingent processes and practices by which differences are produced and encoded in clinical knowledges and in broader sociohistorical identities.

The final part of this book, "Dislocations," further unhinges the production of difference from the local and resituates it within translocal connectivities. In this set of chapters I rethink some of the key tropes—kinship, for example—in anthropological studies of China, Chinese diasporas, and Chinese medicine, and I examine how dualistic discourses of "East" and "West," "culture" and "science," "tradition" and "modernity," and "local" and "global" are repeatedly invoked and deployed in the everydayness of Chinese medicine. I contend that these tropes are the outcomes—rather than explanations—of particular kinds of translocal encounters of traditional Chinese medicine. As I examine the ways in which "kinship," "culture," "China," and "America" come to life in everyday practice, I move toward an analysis of plurality and contingency in the production of difference, as well as an understanding of how specific spatiotemporalities emerge through practices of mapping, temporalizing, and positioning.

Chapter 5, "Engendering Families and Knowledges, Sideways," examines a seemingly archaic mode of knowledge production in Chinese medicine—namely, the transmission of knowledge through kinship ties in general and patrilineal descent in particular. Rather than focus on men as the protagonists among knowledge bearers, I discuss the life histories of three Chinese women who entered or left Chinese medicine through kinship ties. I refocus the question of gender and kinship in Chinese medicine and then turn it sideways to examine the translocal production of difference through family ties, claims to knowledges and identities, and authorities over knowledges. Discourses and practices of kinship and gender in Chinese medicine are as much about continuity and connection as they are about the rupture and alienation that continue to shape the worlding of Chinese medicine.

In chapter 6, "Discrepant Distances," I focus on my ethnographic encounters in the San Francisco Bay Area in order to discuss the ways in which the distances between "China" and "America" are measured through the worlding of Chinese medicine. I examine how translocal encounters do not produce a uniform transpacific community of traditional Chinese medicine but instead provide occasions for making strategic alliances and, at the same time, reproduce and transform existing terms of differences. Whereas "America" occupies an intimate place in China's imaginaries of the world, "China" seems distant in time and space to many non-Chinese practitioners of Chinese medicine. Even though the "Chinese century" may seem more imminent and inevitable than ever as the end of the first decade of the new millennium draws near, "China" remains a shifting and elusive sign at once close and unreachable, familiar and alien, backward and too far ahead.

Part One

ENTANGLEMENTS

One

GET ON
TRACK
WITH THE
WORLD

"Cynthia," the name by which she was known to foreign students and trainees, was an acupuncturist at the Shuguang Hospital of Traditional Chinese Medicine in Shanghai. She was less known for her medical expertise, however, than for being an avid reader of newspapers. She was not a big follower of headline news—whether it was about the reforms to reduce or even eliminate state subsidies of healthcare, or about the structural unemployment that swept across state-owned enterprises at the end of the 1990s. Instead, her focus was the newspaper's real estate section, and the advertisements of upscale residences were her passion. Cynthia was getting married, and she wanted to buy a home.[1]

It came as little surprise, then, that the most engaging conversation I ever had with Cynthia was not about traditional Chinese medicine but about homes in Palo Alto, California. A few days after that conversation she showed me a newspaper advertisement of her dream home, Jinqiu California Garden, a gated community of luxury condos developed by a Hong Kong real estate company in the suburb of Shanghai. Cynthia read the advertisement out loud to me: "Jinqiu California Garden offers you a California-style living space, as well as a healthy, wealthy, elegant lifestyle. As part of our 1999 Lunar New Year's special events, we offer our homeowners a one-day free clinic where they can consult famous traditional doctors about health problems." Turning to me, she said, "California lifestyle and traditional Chinese medicine—what a strange combination! But I'd love to be their resident acupuncturist!"

What makes the production of a healthy, wealthy lifestyle, crystallized in an imagined California, an effective marketing strategy in Shanghai's real estate market? At first glance this question points in the direction of global connections and imaginations that not only extend well beyond the city of Shanghai but also seem to elude the boundary of the nation-state. However, the phenomenon of Jinqiu California Garden, both in its marketing strategy and its market allure, cannot simply be explained as a case in which the local is penetrated by, absorbed into, and thereby reconstituted by global capitalism: after all, how do we explain why California in particular sells in Shanghai? More strikingly, why does the inclusion of a traditional Chinese medicine clinic, which is a highly unusual feature in Shanghai's residential neighborhood, add to and even authenticate Jinqiu California Garden's "California" appeal?

Contrary to Cynthia's view, those who have lived in California in the past twenty years probably would not find acupuncture and herbal medicine, the two main components of traditional Chinese medicine, completely alien concepts and practices. Indeed, when I tell friends in the San Francisco Bay Area about my research on traditional Chinese medicine, many of them eagerly tell me, "You should interview *my* acupuncturist!" The popularity of traditional Chinese medicine is also reflected in and produced through mass media across the United States. In the last two decades, images and discussions of acupuncture and herbal medicine have been seen in magazines ranging from *Esquire* to the *Harvard Magazine.* The popular men's magazine *Esquire,* for example, featured the actor David Duchovny from the television sci-fi series *The X-Files* on the cover of its May 1999 issue. In *The X-Files* Duchovny plays an FBI agent who dedicates his life to the pursuit of space aliens and other paranormal phenomena. The cover of the magazine sported an image of Duchovny adorned with acupuncture needles protruding from head and face—under which the caption read "David Duchovny's Death-Defying Acts." Traditional Chinese medicine and other forms of complementary and alternative medicines have received just as much if not more attention from popular media in the San Francisco Bay Area. The March 1997 issue of the magazine *San Francisco Focus* featured on its front cover an image of a regular plastic prescription

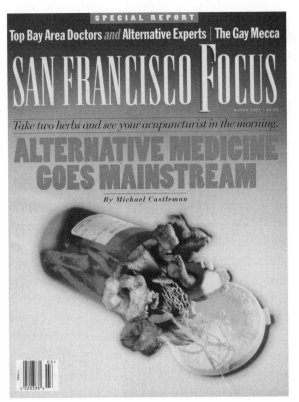

The cover of *San Francisco Focus*, March 1997. Courtesy *San Francisco* magazine.

bottle with its cap off, out of which spilled ginseng, ganoderma lucidum (*lingzhi*), astragalus membranaceus (*huangqi*) and a variety of other Chinese herbs. Above this striking image was the sensational title of a special report: "Take Two Herbs and See Your Acupuncturist in the Morning: Alternative Medicine Goes Mainstream."

The images and anecdotes offered above provide a window onto translocal formations that are more imaginative and effervescent than what can be subsumed under the umbrella of globalization. They call for ethnographic and analytical strategies that do not assume a priori a singular "global era" within which the ethnographies of local lives and translocal movements are to take place. Instead, they point toward ways in which differences are produced *through*—rather than *in spite of*—cosmopolitan aspirations and global ambitions. In this chapter I begin to introduce an ethnographic analysis of how traditional Chinese medicine is made and remade through multi-sited, multidirectional, and sociohistorically contingent projects and processes that also produce visions, understandings, and experiences of racialized, class-girded worlds. To do so, I focus on two historical moments in the worlding of traditional Chinese medicine: the first moment took place from the 1960s to the early 1970s and the second from the 1990s to the present. I chose these two moments to highlight the discrepant world-making projects that not only shape the worlds we inhabit but also challenge any uniform, abstract, or transcendental sense of global spatiotemporality.

Cosmopolitan Aspirations

From the 1960s to early 1970s, during the cold war era, the Chinese government organized the export of traditional Chinese medicine as a quintessentially Chinese, low-cost, low-tech, preventive medicine suitable for healthcare in Third World countries, especially those in Africa. The proliferation of traditional Chinese medicine as a preventive medicine for the rural poor helped envision and produce a "proletariat world" that China strove to champion. Beginning in the early 1980s, however, this traveling route of traditional Chinese medicine—as well as the vision and salience of the proletariat world—was eclipsed by other routes and worlds. By the 1990s, as China continued its economic and social reforms to "get on track with the world" (*yu shijie jiegui*), the transnational trafficking of traditional Chinese medicine would take place most intensively between China and North America, Europe, and East Asia. Meanwhile in the Bay Area and in California more broadly, traditional Chinese medicine as a naturalistic, preventive medicine has evolved out of Chinatown and departed from its counterculture trajectories of the 1960s. Today it is a mainstream, urban, middle-class practice, deeply enmeshed in the commodification and consumption of health and medicine (see chapter 2).

Shanghai-based practitioners become aware of this shift in preventive medicine through transnational travel encounters, professional journals, mass media, and new information technology. In clinical practices and in everyday life, they forge new professional and social alliances and networks in reinventing traditional Chinese medicine as a new kind of preventive medicine. They do so by locating traditional Chinese medicine at the cutting edge of modern medical science and an emerging "cosmopolitan medicine," and by associating the consumption of traditional Chinese medicine with a middle-class lifestyle. This entails redefining the scope of health conditions on which traditional Chinese medicine focuses, as well as fashioning a particular clientele at home and abroad—an emerging middle class that aspires to be "white." In particular, practitioners and entrepreneurs of traditional Chinese medicine have invented a new medical concept called "subhealth" (*yajiankang*) to characterize the state of health of the urban and, especially, young middle class. Within this context it is not so paradoxical, after all, that the inclusion of a traditional Chinese medicine clinic within a gated community should accentuate the latter's appeal as a California-style, upper-middle-class living space in Shanghai.

In the pages that follow I navigate a journey that goes back and forth between China and Africa, Shanghai and San Francisco. In doing so, I highlight the discrepant cosmopolitan dreams and aspirations that have produced specific kinds of knowledges, patterns of difference and solidarity, and particular spatiotemporalities of emergent worlds. As Aihwa Ong and Donald Nonini (1997:12) point out, much of the literature on late capitalism and postmodernity is limited to Euro-American societies and thus runs the risk of taking particular social formations and experiences as universal. Ong and Nonini instead trace what they call an Asia-Pacific "Chinese transnationalism"—the historical roots of which reach back into the eighteenth century. Centering around diasporic Chinese communities, this "ungrounded empire" also encounters various forms and narratives of nation, capitalism, modernity, and cosmopolitanism. Yet in spite of its encounters with "global capital," Chinese transnationalism remains a "distinctive postcolonial formation" and "a culturally distinctive domain" (4). I find this analysis important for finding alternatives to the Euro-American–centered view of late capitalism, as well as demonstrative of how the deployment of Chineseness can be a strategic intervention in the universalistic discourse of globalization.

Like Ong and Nonini, I am interested in exploring alternative forms of globalization and cosmopolitanism. I am less invested, however, in Chinese cosmopolitanism as a culturally distinctive alternative to Euro-American-centric global configurations. Rather, I focus on how specific forms of cosmopolitanism emerge through uneven translocal relations that require the rethinking of what counts as local and what counts as global. In reviewing the history of cosmopolitanism and colonialism in Southeast Asia, Pheng Cheah (2006) identifies two types of Chinese cosmopolitanism: a mercantilist cosmopolitanism that is promoted by European colonial policies but misread as Confucianism; and a fiercely patriotic and revolutionary cosmopolitanism that, having contributed to Chinese nationalism and anticolonial struggles around the opening of the twentieth century, is now invoked by the Chinese state to attract overseas capital and expertise. Rather than rely on cultural distinction, Cheah questions the singularity and Chinese-ness of Chinese cosmopolitanism by exploring cosmopolitanisms as situated and transformative historical formations. Just as attentive to translocal fields of power but with an emphasis on China's new cosmopolitan projects, Lisa Rofel (2007) coins the phrase "cosmopolitanism with Chinese characteristics" that foregrounds the "self-conscious transcendence of locality, and the domestication of the world by way of renegotiating China's position in the world" (111). The reinvention of China entails a reinvention of the world. These discussions bring into focus that, first, the distinctiveness of Chinese cosmopolitanisms has less to do with cultural logic or essence than it does with the contingent outcome of specific translocal power fields. Second, the global figures in cosmopolitan imaginaries serve as a point of reference rather than a ready-made overarching framework. It follows that, third, cosmopolitanisms are grounded in, and in turn reproduce and transform, particular forms of disparities and differences. In light of these critical reflections on Chinese cosmopolitanisms, my aim here is to examine how shifting terms of difference—especially the deployment of race and class—are embedded and articulated through various cosmopolitan, world-making projects. The worlding of Chinese medicine conjures cosmopolitan dreams and aspirations from disparate locations. In so doing it promises the transcendence of locality and yet remains deeply entangled in discourses of race and class that render these aspirations anything but transcendental—be it Jinqiu California Garden or the proletariat world that Chinese medicine was to serve.

"Serve the People of the World"

On August 7, 1950, at the first National Conference of Health of the newly founded People's Republic of China, Mao Zedong declared that China's healthcare policy should "serve workers, peasants, and soldiers, focus on prevention, and promote the solidarity of Chinese and Western medicines."[2] These words were soon turned into China's official healthcare policies. In their implementation, these policies emphasized combining basic biomedical and traditional Chinese medical practices for the prevention of infectious diseases afflicting the working people and for an inclusive coverage of healthcare. In June 26, 1965, on the eve of the Cultural Revolution (1966–76), Mao further declared that China's healthcare should focus on poor peasants in rural China, to whom biomedicine remained largely unavailable in spite of the dominance of biomedical hospitals in large cities. In China this new declaration is referred to simply as the "6.26 Instruction."

These policies had a profound impact on the practice of traditional Chinese medicine. First, beginning in 1956, by adopting the institutional, pedagogical, and clinical standards of biomedicine, state-run traditional Chinese medicine colleges and hospitals came to replace family clinics and small academies (Farquhar 1994; Leslie 1977; Taylor 2005). At the same time, local priests and itinerant healers were ordered to abandon their "superstitious" or "unprofessional" practices and thus were excluded from the official version of traditional Chinese medicine.

Moreover, even though Mao declared in 1954 that traditional Chinese medicine is "our motherland's treasure house," many Chinese—especially urban Chinese—still saw it as backward and inferior to biomedicine. A state-initiated campaign to scientize traditional Chinese medicine lasted through the 1960s. A *People's Daily* editorial on October 20, 1954, spelled out the content of this campaign. Its immediate goal was to develop a body of basic theories that could then be rectified by scientific methods, especially through experiments. At a broader level, traditional Chinese medicine was posited as a quintessentially "Chinese science" that was distinctive from "Western science" and needed to be integrated into modern science and medicine. According to the editorial, traditional Chinese medicine should play "a supplementary role" in modern medicine and that this modern medicine "should reflect the uniqueness of China's geography and climate, the uniqueness of Chinese herbs and their applications, and the uniqueness of the life and work of the Chinese of all ethnicities." Yet, the editorial continues, because traditional Chinese medicine truly is science, albeit a Chinese science, it deserved to be universalized and shared by the world.

What did the world look like then? As part of the cold war geopolitics China, the United States, and the Soviet Union were all sending aid, including medical aid, to Africa, Latin America, and the developing countries in Asia (Eadie and Grizzell 1979; Hutchison 1975; Larkin 1971). In crafting a distinctive geopolitical niche for China, the Chinese state fashioned a world that was epitomized in the construction of an "international proletariat," and it was this world that China strove to lead. As part of its world-making effort, the Chinese government exported a kind of "preventive medicine" formed of a mixture of biomedicine and acupuncture, which was similar to what was practiced in rural China at the time. According to Elisabeth Hsu

(2007), Chinese medical teams typically consisted of nine to ten biomedical professionals and one acupuncturist. Compared to its railway projects in Africa, as well as its agricultural aid and other economic aid to the area, China's medical aid was one of the most successful forms of aid precisely because it targeted rural and disaster areas (Hutchison 1975; Larkin 1971; Snow 1988). According to a survey by Gail Eadie and Denise Grizzell (1979), Chinese medical teams were ubiquitous in Third World countries, especially Afria. In 1976 alone they were in sixteen countries. In China it was common to read Chinese newspaper articles that applauded the medical miracles that Chinese medical teams produced in Somalia, Algeria, Mauritania, and other African countries (see *People's Daily* 1966, 1967, 1970).

On February 10, 1970, the *People's Daily* published an article titled "Serve the People of Mauritania." The article recounted heroic stories where the Chinese medical team produced various kinds of medical miracles, including delivering a baby for a young peasant couple under unthinkable conditions; removing a fifteen-kilogram ovarian tumor from a poor nomad woman; and improvising antibiotic drugs. In a style typical of news reports and propaganda of the time, the nomad woman was quoted to have said, "Chairman Mao gave me a second life. I'll never forget Chairman Mao. Long live Chairman Mao!"

Acupuncture was the most captivating feature that distinguished the Chinese medical teams from other teams and "aroused interest throughout Africa" (Hutchison 1975:222). In Zanzibar acupuncture was held in such high esteem that those with a bad temper were told to take it to the Chinese because "they even have a cure for that." In Mauritania, the Chinese trained the first native acupuncturist—a local young nurse. After apprenticing with the Chinese acupuncturists he was able to treat various pains by needling more than sixty acupuncture points. As he exclaimed, "Chinese acupuncture is particularly useful in our country, where there is a lack of doctors and medicine" (*People's Daily* 1970:5). By the end of the 1970s, acupuncture was employed in hospitals across Africa and was sometimes performed by locals. Acupuncture anesthesia was used in surgical procedures such as caesarian birth and tumor removal (Eadie and Grizzell 1979:229).

The image of an international proletariat was thus embodied in the worlding of traditional Chinese medicine as a low-cost and low-tech preventive medicine perfect for the poor and underprivileged of Africa. Here the notion of class was doubly encoded—in the alliance of China and Africa as both part of the "Third World," and in the fact that the Chinese medical team served poor peasants and nomads. The emphasis on peasantry merits particular attention. As Ann Anagnost (1997:23) has argued, in the 1950s and 1960s—through the body of the oppressed, suffering peasant subject—Maoist ideology recast into Marxian class opposition and struggle the inequalities internal to Chinese society, and then made these inequalities continuous with China's subaltern status in a world of nation-states. Anagnost also notes that in contrast to the classic Marxist theory that depicted peasantry as the dead-weight lumpenproletariat, the Chinese state represented poor peasants and nomads (*nongmu min*) as the most revolutionary of all proletariats because they suffered the most (30; cf. Marx 1852). I further argue here that China's international "subaltern status" itself was also produced by the worlding of this particular configuration and representation of the proletariat—one that was not overdetermined by Marxian universals but instead mediated through the carefully crafted body of the global peasant.

Moreover, the centrality of Africa in the production of the international proletariat was compounded by the racialization of class. In a widely quoted speech Mao claimed that "in Africa, in Asia, in every part of the world there is racism; in reality, racial problems are class problems" *(People's Daily* 1963:1, quoted in Dikötter 1992:192).[3] The Chinese state went as far as striving to construct a common racialized identity across China and Africa, urging that "we blacks stick together" against the "white race" (Hutchison 1975:179).[4] In practice, China treated the whole continent as a more or less homogenous area diplomatically and administratively, at the same time stressing that China and Africa shared a common history of racial and colonial oppression as well as centuries-old trade and cultural links.

I do not suggest that "race" or "class" serves a stable, real scheme of classification. Rather, as Judith Butler (2000) has argued, "race" and "class" are invoked and appropriated as contingent points of reference in the production of differences. This racialized and class-girded proletariat world was also re-created back in China through the worlding of traditional Chinese medicine. In 1974, China and the WHO cofounded the International Acupuncture Training Center at the Shanghai College of Traditional Chinese medicine (SCTCM). The first class consisted of twelve students from eleven countries (ten African countries and Laos) (Shi 1997:782), and the WHO and the Chinese government funded all of the students. The proletariat world, and China's engagement with Africa in building that world, was no mere fantasy: it was the votes by the African nation-states in

1970 that tipped the balance and allowed the People's Republic of China to become a member of the United Nations.

However, the world of the international proletariat was not readily embraced and enacted by all. Even those who participated in the worlding of Chinese medicine had doubts about the racialized proletariat brotherhood. On the one hand many African students complained about racial discrimination during their stay in China (Snow 1988). On the other hand their Chinese hosts also articulated ambivalences toward African students. Many of the senior acupuncturists and herbal doctors put in charge of training international students attended SCTCM in the 1950s. The majority of them came from middle-class *zhishifenzi* (intelligentsia) backgrounds, some from families that had had successful businesses in traditional Chinese medicine for generations. They did not always share revolutionary "proletariat" sentiments. During the Cultural Revolution, groups of Red Guards—many of whom were students at SCTCM and nearby high schools—and local factory workers took over the administration and in some cases clinical practice at the college and its teaching hospitals. Senior practitioners were marginalized and their professional authority subverted to the extent that a few leading figures in traditional Chinese medicine were persecuted to death (*pohai zhisi*), driven to suicide (*Shanghai Kangfu Zazhi* 1989). Senior practitioners who were allowed to train African students did so under the watchful eyes of factory workers and Red Guards. When recounting their experiences to me, these practitioners accentuated feelings of alienation toward their African students as well as Chinese workers and Red Guards.

These practitioners were also the first to notice a marked change in the composition of their overseas students. In the 1980s, they began to see more and more self-funded students from East Asia, Europe, and North America. Indeed, at SCTCM beginning in 1983, the number of international students sponsored by WHO and the government decreased each year. Meanwhile, SCTCM started admitting self-funded foreign students and trainees, most of whom came from Europe, North America, and East Asia. In 1994, for example, SUTCM and its teaching hospitals were visited by 328 overseas acupuncture students, trainees, and observers who hailed from a diverse group of countries including Japan, Korea, Britain, Germany, France, Iran, Denmark, Italy, Austria, Belgium, Colombia, Australia, Canada, and the United States (Shi 1997:783).

The changes in the nationalities and funding of international students are indicative of broader sociohistorical shifts in the experiences, under-

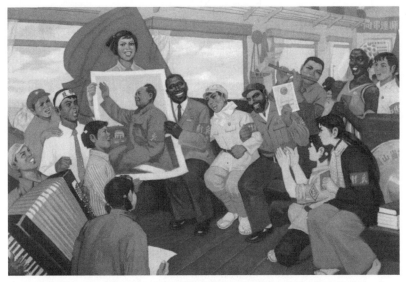

A propaganda poster during the Cultural Revolution depicting the happy members of a proletariat world riding together on a train. Poster courtesy of Susan Greenhalgh.

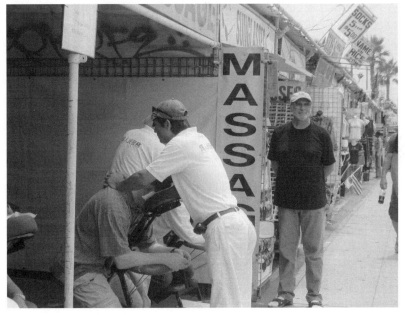

A massage (*tuina*) shop in Venice Beach, California. The workers wear shirts inscribed with the Chinese characters "Serve the people." Photo by the author.

standings, and practices of what makes up the world. Specifically, in the reform era, the place of Africa on China's map of the world has been eclipsed by affluent nations in North America, Europe, and East Asia. Although Africa epitomized the international proletariat that Maoist China claimed to champion, in the 1990s Africa was reimagined to be the undesirable land of poverty and backwardness. This spatial realignment is crystallized in the construction of a world that is middle class and "white." As one administrator at SUTCM said to me with undisguised excitement, "This year [1999] we are getting a lot of students from the United States, not just Japan and Korea, to join our four-year regular college program. These students are not overseas Chinese either. They are white! Finally, we've become *truly* international!"

The administrator's blunt remarks bring to the fore a reinvented past configured as backward and isolated, as well as a present in which imagined whiteness marks a "truly" international space with which China strives to get on track. This reracialized idea of the "international" is also reflected in the experiences of some—though not all—Asian American students who go to China to study Chinese medicine. I first met David Luo, a young biomedical physician who practices in San Francisco, at the International Acupuncture Training Program at SUTCM in 1999. He and a number of other Chinese American students complained to me that they were treated differently from their white colleagues. David told me in an interview that, during a publicity photo session with their teacher at one of the SUTCM teaching hospitals, he and another student of Asian descent were pushed aside so that a blond woman could be next to the teacher in the picture. Race and class have not disappeared in contemporary discourses of traditional Chinese medicine but instead have been refigured. In this case, being international has become conflated with whiteness: whereas Africanness stands for undesirable kinds of internationalism, Asian Americans are seen as not international enough. In sum, aspirations to transcend are decidedly not transcendental.

"Get on Track with the World"

Shanghai did not emerge as a cosmopolitan urban center, let alone the "Paris of the Orient," until it was made a treaty port at the end of the first Opium War (1839–1842). During my childhood and adolescent years in Shanghai I often heard my parents and their friends, especially those visiting from out of town, lightheartedly describe various aspects of life in

Shanghai as being *haipai,* or "Shanghai-style." For these friends, for example, haipai Peking opera was crowd-pleasing, westernized, and unorthodox. Haipai cuisine was quick to absorb the latest trends in various culinary traditions (both inside and outside of China) and for the most part was easy on the palate, although it suffered from the lack of a distinctive regional character. The kind of Chinese medicine taught and practiced at SUTCM was not exempt from the haipai label. Known for its strength in the biomedical components of the curriculum, clinical practice, and laboratory and clinical research—especially compared with other colleges of traditional Chinese medicine in China and abroad—SUTCM earned a haipai reputation among admirers and critics alike. Intimately linked with Shanghai's entanglements in its colonial past as well as with China's future, haipai signals for the Shanghainese a cultivated and studied indifference to cultural imports as well as a hyperawareness of their own enmeshment in worlds in the making. When invoked by critics, however, haipai comes to stand for the absence of purity and authenticity and an all-too-ready embracement of the outside and the new.

In the 1990s haipai again became a buzzword. A 1999 poll in Shanghai showed that one of the most popular new expressions of the year was for China to "get on track with the world" (*yu shijie jiegui*), a slogan that was first initiated by the central government but then quickly gained popularity in everyday discourse. But to say that China *needed* to get on track with the world indexes the anxiety many Chinese felt that, at the end of the 1990s, China was still not quite part of the world. How could this be? To begin, the world that China strives to get on track with now is distinctively different from the 1960s world charted out through the worlding of traditional Chinese medicine. The cold war era has come to an end. Central and local governments have been pursuing economic and social reforms to produce a transnational market economy that promises to bring prosperity to China.

Shanghai again sees itself at the forefront of these new geopolitical, economic, and social trends. During my fieldwork I was struck by the fact that when discussing their conceptions of the ideal world, Shanghainese from every walk of life often referred specifically to the United States and Europe to convey their thoughts on "how things could improve in China," and how China should position itself in relation to the world. These references were often articulated in complex and sometimes contradictory ways.

To get on track with the world, then, means more than simply opening up and reaching out—it entails constructing a particular kind of world at home. In the everyday life of the Shanghainese, this begins with imagining and fashioning a universalistic middle-class consumption pattern and lifestyle in the image of the white middle class of the United States and of the European Union. In particular, government policies since the 1980s have channeled a large portion of individual expenditure into private home purchasing, healthcare, and higher education.

The shifts in healthcare practices are marked by the dismantling of the socialist welfare system and the privatization of health insurance. In the early 1990s a council was set up within the Shanghai municipal government to embark on the privatization of healthcare (Shanghai Medical Insurance Bureau 1998). As an official at the Shanghai Medical Insurance Bureau told me:

> Healthcare was part of the socialist state welfare system. An employee was part of their work unit all their life. That was a fixed relationship. The work unit covered the worker's medical expenses—the same way that it also allocated housing. Now we are moving toward a market economy and we need a labor market, which means we also need a flexible labor force. So we want a more flexible health insurance system where the state, the enterprise, and the individual share the cost of healthcare. That's just part of market economy.
>
> We took field trips to the United States, Germany, Singapore, and other countries to learn from their medial insurance policies. We cannot afford the U.S. system—it's too commercialized. But we found the German and Singaporean models, where the state collects a premium, more realistic for us.

Under the reform plan proposed in November 1998, Shanghai's medical insurance would be primarily financed through contributions from local enterprises, including state-owned and collective-owned enterprises, joint ventures, foreign ventures, and private businesses. Employees would pay a total premium of 7.5 percent of their monthly salaries (Shanghai Medical Insurance Bureau 1998). The reform was first implemented among retirees on November 1, 1998. The privatization of healthcare favored the emerging middle class, many of whom worked for multinational or private companies. However, it added to the financial strains on the workers at state-owned enterprises, whose income and job security were on the line as these enterprises experienced sharp declines in revenues and even bankruptcy at the end of the 1990s.

Against this background, the Shanghainese have seen the emergence of a new, naturalistic preventive health concept and practice that bears strikingly little resemblance to the kind of preventive medicine worlded during the Mao era. This new preventive medicine mainly targets the chronic illnesses associated with urban middle-class lifestyles, and stresses long-term overall well-being. If this sounds familiar to Californians, it is probably because California has indeed been a key player in the production of the new preventive medicine as well as in the worlding of traditional Chinese medicine in the 1990s. In the following section I describe the changing trajectories of traditional Chinese medicine in California, as well as how the practice and discourse of traditional Chinese medicine has transformed the biomedical mainstream.

Reinventing Traditional Chinese Medicine in California

What has happened in medicine in California? Until the mid-twentieth century acupuncture and herbal medicine were mainly practiced behind closed doors in small Chinese American communities.[5] In the 1960s the counterculture movement recast traditional Chinese medicine as a naturalistic and holistic alternative to the biomedical establishment. After James Reston's trip to China in July 1971 and his dramatic encounter with acupuncture, in the United States a frenzy over Chinese medicine quickly swept through the scientific and biomedical communities as well as the tiny but resilient community of traditional Chinese medical practitioners (see the introduction). Delegations of research scientists and biomedical professionals went to China to study acupuncture and herbal medicine, and soon thereafter started publishing field reports and research articles on those subjects (American Anesthesia Study Group 1976; American Herbal Pharmacology Delegation 1975).

In California acupuncturists, patient groups, and politicians began joining efforts in campaigning for the legalization of acupuncture. With the passage of California Senate Bill 86 in 1975, California became the fourth U.S. state to legalize acupuncture. However, at the time of its legalization in California, acupuncture still could not be performed without prior diagnosis or referral by a "physician." It was not until 1997 that Senate Bill 212 finally included "acupuncturist" within the definition of "physician" and placed acupuncture within the coverage of worker's compensation. The main force behind the legalization of acupuncture was the powerful alliance between acupuncturists, patients, and politicians and legislators. For

instance, the iconic and charismatic George Moscone, a progressive, Dem-
ocratic state senator who went on to become the mayor of San Francisco
(1976–1978) and whose assassination in 1978 remains one of the most sensational events in the history of the city, is still admired today by the acupuncture community as a key figure in the campaign.

Yet these alliances were also fragile and crosscut by fissures. As Linda
Barnes (1995, 2005) argued, the mainstreaming of acupuncture and traditional Chinese medicine in the United States has taken place in a racialized framework in which early immigrant practitioners were discriminated
against on the basis of their racial profiles whereas today's white practitioners feel no qualms in claiming a place in the world of traditional Chinese medicine. Although California is becoming increasingly ethnically
diverse, the ethnic composition of traditional Chinese medicine practitioners has instead bifurcated.[6] In the absence of official statistics, leaders of
traditional Chinese medicine organizations in California estimate that over
50 percent of practitioners of acupuncture in California are of Caucasian
descent, and the rest consist mainly of those of East Asian descent such as
Chinese, Korean, Vietnamese, and Japanese. In the Bay Area colleges of traditional Chinese medicine, students who enter under the category "white,
non-Hispanic" take up 60 percent (and sometimes much more) of the
enrollment.[7]

During my fieldwork I encountered quite a few projects by various local acupuncture associations and groups—often roughly drawn along the
lines of ethnic groups, educational backgrounds, and immigration histories. Each of these projects presented its own account of the early years of
struggles, and the resulting histories and memoirs were rich in invaluable
information and personal accounts and thus were witness to a passionate
and definitive era. However, even though there was much consensus over
the key events leading to the legalization and subsequent legislature of acupuncture, the authors and sponsors of the projects often disagreed over the
specific contribution of a group or an individual, and consensus building
took painstaking negotiations.[8] I do not intend to reduce these disagree-
ments to simple racial politics. What I do suggest is that a wide range of
activist groups from discrepant sociohistorical trajectories and locations—
recent immigrants from mainland China, older immigrants from Hong
Kong, Taiwan, and other parts of East and Southeast Asia, senior acupuncturists trained in the United States or Europe who mostly self-identified as

Caucasian, and so on—experience, approach, and remember the history of legalization in specific, meaningful, and contestatory ways.

By the first decade of the twenty-first century, there were more than six thousand licensed acupuncturists in California authorized by the state to practice acupuncture and prescribe herbs (Dower 2003). In addition, a number of leading insurance companies now provide coverage for acupuncture; hospitals in the Bay Area and elsewhere are beginning to offer services in traditional Chinese medicine; and medical schools are including acupuncture and other CAM therapies within their curricula.[9]

As part of the efforts to broaden the appeal of Chinese medicine as well as their own clinical practice, some acupuncturists in the Bay Area sought out white patient populations. Yuen Chau, an activist and well-known practitioner of traditional Chinese medicine who has worked in San Francisco for more than twenty-five years, not only orients his practice toward white patients but has also moved his family into a white, middle-class neighborhood. As one who was brought up in a family that had practiced acupuncture and herbal medicine in south China for generations, and who then was educated at a well-respected traditional Chinese medicine college in China, Chau prefers being addressed as "Doctor" (*yisheng*). I interviewed him in his clinic on the second floor of a Victorian house in Noe Valley, San Francisco, a predominantly white, upper-middle-class neighborhood. An initial office visit to Chau's clinic costs $45 and the follow-up visits are $10 each. Dr. Chau charges $65 for an acupuncture treatment session, and additional payments for herbal tea. These fees are about average among acupuncturists in the Bay Area. As Dr. Chau stated in our interview:

> Chinese medicine first came to the West Coast when the migrant railroad workers came here in the nineteenth century. I, and many others, came here in the early 1980s. These days the ethnic composition of practitioners in the Bay Area is really diverse. But I can tell you that my patients are 95 percent white. So we've come a long way from the old days when we practiced in Chinatown and served the Chinese populations. All my students are white, except for a few Chinese Americans from Berkeley. I've kept track of my students since twenty-three years ago, when I first started practicing. Among my former patients, 114 became interested in Chinese medicine and started studying it. Some of them went to local traditional Chinese medicine colleges, some went to China, and many apprenticed with me. . . . If traditional Chinese

medicine wants to be accepted by mainstream society, it has to appeal to the white middle class.

Dr. Chau is acutely (and perhaps a bit painfully as well) aware that the demographic majority of California does not automatically become the "mainstream," as what counts as the mainstream is deeply embedded in power-laden configurations and discourses of race, ethnicity, and class. He is not alone in his assessment of the racialized mainstream in California. Although not all acupuncturists deliberately seek out white patients, many of those I interviewed, with the exception of those who work within predominantly ethnic Chinese neighborhoods such as Chinatown and the Sunset District, claim that 85 to 90 percent of their patients are white. According to Veronica Nelson, a physician who has been training with a Chinese herbalist, most of the patients are "between the ages of twenty-five and forty, white, upper-middle class. Those are the patients who have the money and smarts to seek acupuncture."

Corporatizing Cosmopolitan Medicine

Sometimes it is not patients but corporations that have the "money and smarts" to seek out alternative therapies. Dr. Chu Huangsheng, who had a clinic in the South Bay, was well aware of the corporate demand for acupuncture and herbal medicine. With this in mind he advertised his practice on the Internet—an effort that proved successful. On a glorious day in spring 2000 Chu and I went to a company in Silicon Valley that specialized in space technology. On entering the gate we followed the signs that read "health fair vendors" and parked the car. A security guard came over to help, and seeing the acupuncture anatomical model I was carrying he said, "You must be the acupuncturists!"

The health fair ran from 9:00 AM to 2:00 PM. Although most of the booths were conveniently located on the lawn of the cafeteria, Chu's spot was in a room on the side. By the time we arrived several other vendors had set up their booths. Among them was Magnabloc, which in a continuously running video introduced its magnets designed for pain and stress relief—a product that was marketed as the only one of its kind designed by a "physician." A company named Total Health Concept occupied another booth, in which a muscular young man and a sexy young woman with a Spanish accent stood behind a folding treatment table and a machine used to measure "body composition profiles," including water and fat ratios. At a nutrition counter set up in another booth, a man, whose business cards on display testified that he was an M.D., tested visitors for carpal tunnel syndrome and gave out free nutritional advice. Over the counter a banner read: "Do you have the following symptoms? Fatigue, headache and migraine, stress, depression, insomnia. . . . If you do, you should be consulting a nutritionist." Aetna, a health insurance company, gave out free blood pressure screenings. A Japanese woman in a tie-dyed cotton outfit came over from her booth across the room and introduced herself to us. She said that she practices Jin Shin Jyutsu, a Japanese therapy used to improve health by massaging certain points on the body. She asked Chu if he knew about Jin Shin Jyutsu, and he replied that he did, adding: "It's very similar to acupressure."

I helped Chu set up his booth. He brought in a big cardboard sign on which the red characters of the name of his clinic were written against a white background. He propped it up on the table. On one end of the table we set up a male anatomical acupuncture model as well as auricular, hand, and foot acupuncture models. Next to the models were bottles of Chinese formula medicines (*zhongchengyao*). The names were written out both in Chinese characters and in the pinyin romanization system. Classified as food supplements by the FDA, the therapeutic functions of the medicines were not indicated on the bottles. Next to the bottles were boxes of ginseng extracts. On the far end of the table were glass jars of dried Chinese herbs. The name of each herb was written out in both Chinese and Latin, along with its properties according to traditional Chinese medicine. In front of the glass jars was a plastic business card rack in which Chu displayed business cards for himself, his wife, his son, his daughter-in-law, and a chiropractor who practiced at his family clinic.

A middle-aged white man wearing a company nametag around his neck approached us, explaining that he was previewing what would be available at the health fair. His preview turned out to last almost an hour, which made me uncomfortable—the recent Wen Ho Lee "spy case" in which a Taiwanese-born U.S. physicist was accused of stealing nuclear secrets for China was still very much on everybody's mind. Our visitor claimed that he was an advocate of acupuncture and he would seek treatment when he wanted to "tune his body." He said that he was introduced to acupuncture by his wife, and until then he had been very much afraid of the idea of having a needle inserted into his body.

As the lunch hour began, people started wandering into the health fair. I was struck by the highly mixed ethnic and geographical composition of the company employees—Caucasian, African, African American, South Asian, Latino, and East Asian. The most popular booths were the carpal tunnel syndrome testing station and Total Health Concept. At one point there was even a line of about ten people in front of the carpal tunnel station. In the meantime, the Jin Shin Jyutsu practitioner took out her folding bed and treated people on the spot. Chu asked me to hand out packets he had prepared for visitors to his booth. The packet contents included basic information about traditional Chinese medicine and advertisements for his clinic.[10] By 2:00 PM we had distributed about 150 packets. The visitors inquired after a wide range of health problems: diabetes, neck pain, insomnia, post knee nerve surgery treatment, and, of course, carpal tunnel syndrome. Approximately ten visitors had had previous acupuncture treatment, and they asked informed questions such as the difference between acupuncture and chiropractic therapy. Chu explained that in Chinese medicine chiropractic therapy is very similar to *tuina,* or therapeutic massage, and that he even had a chiropractor working at his clinic. The display of raw herbs attracted the most attention, and many of the visitors recognized the ginseng on display.

Chu was also careful to ask the visitors what kind of insurance package they had—the company offered a choice between Kaiser Permanente and Lifeguard. Kaiser did not cover acupuncture unless it was performed by their own physicians, although they were in the process of contracting licensed acupuncturists to work with them. The package offered by Lifeguard, however, included twenty free acupuncture sessions per year. Chu explained that each insurance company offered a different package, and even though it was difficult for an individual to pay an extra premium just to have acupuncture covered by their insurance policy, large corporations had greater resources to cover benefits such as acupuncture.

At the end of the day Diane, one of the organizers of the fair, came to chat with us. She said that this was the seventh year that the company had organized the health fair, but in the first three years they were not able to invite any vendors of alternative medicine because it was not covered by the insurance companies, and the company's Department of Human Relations felt there were issues of liability. By the end of the 1990s, however, things had changed. As Diane stated: "Three years ago, we had a master of *qigong* [a breathing and meditation technique also important in the practice of Chinese martial arts]. He came and he said to everyone who went to see him that he would take away their pain for a day. And the next day everybody was saying that their pain was gone! It was wonderful. I scheduled the fair at lunchtime so that we could get as many people as possible. We posted the event on our intranet [an internal electronic web]. We have about three thousand employees and I think there are six hundred to seven hundred people here today. And we make sure that we have people who do food and diet because that is a huge attraction for employees around lunchtime!"

Beginning in the 1990s, corporations in the Bay Area started to show interest in adding acupuncture and qigong to their benefits package for employees. In practice, these corporations are often concerned with using "preventive" health practices to reduce stress in the corporate environment and to treat health conditions associated with white-collar jobs (see chapter 2). Yet large corporations are not the only groups interested in Chinese medicine as a new kind of "preventive medicine." In 2001, for example, the American Foundation of Traditional Chinese Medicine worked on a project to introduce qigong to the high school curriculum in the San Francisco Unified School District. They succeeded in carrying out short-term pilot programs at a local high school, where students who suffered from depression, anger, and stress reported improvement after practicing simple breathing techniques.

Today in the everyday clinical practice in the Bay Area and across California at large, acupuncture and herbal medicine are primarily used for conditions that are associated with urban lifestyles, and for which biomedicine is less effective or ineffective. A recent national survey indicates that 44 percent of those who use acupuncture do so because conventional biomedical treatments would not help their conditions, whereas 52 percent think that it would be interesting to try (Barnes et al. 2004). These conditions include, for example, allergies and asthma, insomnia, certain pain syndromes, stress and depression, certain types of cancers that are resistant to biomedical therapies, and other chronic illnesses (Barnes et al. 2004; Eisenberg et al. 1993, 1998; National Institutes of Health 1997; Ni et al. 2002). And it is the image of a white, cosmopolitan, middle-class California—and its health problems—that comes to occupy a central place in the worlding of traditional Chinese medicine since the 1990s.

Crafting a World of "Subhealth"

It certainly seems to be no coincidence that the savvy Hong Kong–based developers of Jinqiu California Garden not only recognize the appeal of California in Shanghai's real estate market, but also single out traditional Chinese medicine to authenticate a healthy, wealthy California lifestyle. The marketing strategy of Jinqiu Real Estate Company thus best captures the dreams of an emerging, reracialized middle class that aspires to be cosmopolitan. Like its newspaper advertisement, Jinqiu California Garden's TV infomercial features its one-day traditional Chinese medicine clinic, and focuses the camera on a practitioner who is a twenty-fourth-generation grandson of Li Shizhen (a venerated Ming Dynasty healer). At the end of the infomercial, the CEO of the Jinqiu Real Estate Company tells the audience what this is all about: "The gist of our infomercial is 'go home and enjoy a peaceful, leisurely life.' In a broad sense, this includes . . . having a healthy body. You can't have a healthy mind without a healthy body." In this skillfully crafted infomercial, a cosmopolitan middle-class lifestyle is embodied in the production of a healthy, transnational mind-body. Unlike the view in the 1960s, the kind of "traditional Chinese medicine" we see here is clearly not oriented toward the prevention of infectious diseases among the poor. Nor is it presented as something quintessentially Chinese. Rather, the twenty-fourth-generation grandson of Li Shizhen has been called on to stand for a cosmopolitan preventive medicine that sits comfortably within the image of the California lifestyle.

The rosy picture of traditional Chinese medicine at Jinqiu California Garden, however, should not obscure the fact that health insurance reforms are likely to nudge traditional Chinese medicine into a more marginal, tenuous space within Shanghai's healthcare system. Many practitioners of traditional Chinese medicine worry about the economic impact of the privatization of healthcare, and they do so for a good reason. There are currently over thirty hospitals and research institutes of traditional Chinese medicine in Shanghai. Hospitals in Shanghai, whether biomedical or traditional Chinese, are divided into three groups according to scale, function, and strength in clinical practice and research. Division 1 hospitals are small community hospitals *(jiedao yiyuan)* that serve the neighborhood's basic healthcare needs. Division 2 is made up of larger district-level hospitals *(quji yiyuan)*. Division 3 hospitals, the best equipped and staffed of all three groups, include the teaching hospitals of the three major medical universities in Shanghai: Shanghai Medical University, Shanghai No. 2 Medical University, and the Shanghai University of Traditional Chinese Medicine. The departments and practitioners of traditional Chinese medicine are concentrated in the three teaching hospitals of sUTCM: Shuguang Hospital, Longhua Hospital, and Yueyang Hospital. All three are division 3 hospitals.

The reformed health insurance system allows each individual to choose two designated hospitals that would be covered by their medical insurance: one division 1 hospital, and one division 2 or division 3 hospital. When choosing their designated division 3 hospital, most patients prefer biomedical hospitals for their strength in surgery, biomedical medication, equipment, and their presumed advantage in dealing with "serious illnesses" such as cancer, as well as emergencies. At the same time, patients are more likely to go to a division 1 rather than a traditional Chinese hospital for basic healthcare needs because the former charges lower fees and also tends to be more conveniently located. Practitioners at Shuguang Hospital told me that they began to see a drop in the number of patients beginning at the end of 1998, even though the hospital administration asserted that its statistics had not shown any significant decrease. During my last weeks at Shuguang Hospital I witnessed occasional incidents in which old patients came in apologizing to their doctors for not being able to continue treatment because of changes in their designated healthcare providers. At the end of a slow day, after the departure of the only patient who visited the Department of Internal Medicine that afternoon, a practitioner loudly complained, "Why do we bother to set apart Chinese and Western medicines—the only effect is that we don't even get patients here anymore!"

Healthcare reforms and especially marketization have prompted many practitioners and other proponents of traditional Chinese medicine to search for a new clientele. Some strive to reinvent their practice as a form of preventive medicine for the middle-class, cosmopolitan lifestyle. Li Fengyi, a well-known herbalist born in the 1950s, actively seeks out and even helps construct particular neighborhoods and communities to market his new health concepts and products. In 1994, inspired by Deng Xiaoping's much-publicized speech that promoted private entrepreneurship, Li resigned from his job at Shuguang Hospital and started networking with local and overseas capital to open the Jiren Clinic and Research Institute of Traditional Chinese Medicine—one of the first private clinics in Shanghai.

This enterprise is a multifunctional one where Li and his employees treat patients, train interns, conduct clinical research, and market Li's own Chinese formula medicines. By 2003, his business had expanded into four clinics (all located in downtown Shanghai where the price of real estate had become quite steep) as well as two herbal product factories and eight retail branches in nearby provinces.

Li also travels extensively both within and outside of China. He insists that traveling to North America and Europe has put him in touch with the cutting-edge developments in medicine. And he makes sure that he keeps attuned to the latest trends in medicine by reading up on translated medical literatures. Li's success—which is mediated by, and in turn mediates, the multiple and at times seemingly disparate translocal networks and activities that he engages in—has made him an icon, albeit a somewhat iconoclastic one, of Shanghai's medical circle. Although most of his patients at his private clinic are victims of serious medical conditions such as cancer and liver diseases, the herbal products that he manufactures and markets are decidedly "preventive." Indeed, as I will discuss in greater detail in chapter 3, his success in treating cancer and liver diseases lends credibility and attractiveness to his push for preventive health concepts and products. His colleagues, students, and fans have repeatedly told me that Li has a "vision"—one that would transform traditional Chinese medicine into a naturalistic, preventive, cosmopolitan medicine and locate it at the cutting edge of modern medical science.

To this end, Li and others began exploring a new health concept in the 1990s that they called *yajiankang* ("subhealth"). Although they were not able to state a clear definition of yajiankang, Li and a few other like-minded practitioners of traditional Chinese medicine in Shanghai told me that it indicates a state between being healthy and being ill; that is, it applies to the health conditions of people who, even without any diagnosed or diagnosable disease, suffer from a variety of symptoms such as low energy, fatigue, headaches, insomnia, heart palpitation, and a general sense of being unwell. They further argued that more and more white-collar urban dwellers had become victims of yajiankang, which could lead to chronic illnesses and even premature death. As yajiankang became more and more of a serious issue in Shanghai and other urban centers, it provided a unique niche for Chinese medicine as a "preventive medicine" that focused on the overall bodily constitution and health conditions of the patient and did not rely on the diagnosis of a specific disease in biomedical terms as the precondition for further medical interventions. Curiously, although Li and his colleagues insisted that yajiankang was a concept that they heard about from "foreign medical experts," when I talked to my interlocutors in California in 1999 they told me that they had not heard of the term, even though the description seemed akin to the kinds of conditions they treated routinely.

On a rainy day in September 1998 I caught my first glimpse of the concept of subhealth in operation. Li and others had organized a one-day health fair at a youth center in Hongkou District, a traditionally working-class neighborhood that had recently seen a rapid increase in new, upscale apartment buildings. The health fair, called "Say Good-bye to Sniffles," targeted the prevention and treatment of allergies and asthma. It was cosponsored by SUTCM, the Jiren Clinic and Research Institute of Traditional Chinese Medicine, *Shanghai Popular Health News*, the WHO Center for Health Education and Improvement in Shanghai, and the Shanghai Cancer Recovery Club. Li had told me that he had three goals in mind when he prepared for the health fair: to conduct a survey of the general health condition of the neighborhood residents; to serve their preventive health needs through free health consultations; and to sell Daren Lingzhi, one of his Chinese formula medicines.

I arrived at the health fair at 9:00 AM. Five young women warmly greeted me at the door. They were each wearing a red sash that read "ambassador of compassion." I later found out that they were members of the Cancer Recovery Club and former patients of Li's. Most of them had been laid off from factory jobs in the recent wave of structural unemployment. Li paid them five hundred yuan a month, which was twice the unemployment wage, to help out at health fairs such as this and to go to various neighborhoods to advertise Li's new preventive health concepts and products. Li said that he wanted to help cancer patients through group support, as well as help unemployed women regain their self-esteem.

The health fair took place in the spacious main hall of the youth center. The place was packed in spite of the pouring rain that is typical of the typhoon season. Each visitor was asked to fill out a health survey on entering, and in observing them I noticed that most of the people there were young people under the age of thirty-five, and there were many children accompanied by their parents. This was a surprise to me because the patients I encounter at traditional Chinese medicine clinics and hospitals on an everyday basis are mostly seniors or younger people who are seriously ill. Li later explained to me that he targeted the younger generations because their stressful modern lifestyles make them more susceptible to immune system disorders such as allergies and asthma. His formula medicine Daren Lingzhi, which were capsules of the extract of the large hard, woody fungus *lingzhi*, or ganoderma, was used to tonify *qi* (vital force) and thus strengthen the immune system by raising the T-cell count (Wang et al. 1999).

There were twenty practitioners, all wearing white lab coats, sitting behind desks assembled in a U shape. Li sat facing the entrance in the middle of the U, and I sat next to him. He spent about fifteen minutes with each patient, asking about their health complaints, feeling their pulses, checking the color and texture of their tongues, and giving out relevant advice. Over and over again he told the patients: "You [or your child] work too hard and are too stressed out. You have to learn to take care of yourself. Right now you are only suffering from allergies or asthma. But, in the long run, stress, fatigue, and lack of self-care can destroy your immune system, and that can lead to serious illnesses like cancer, diabetes, and hypertension. Prevention is the key!" Most of the visitors seemed keen to follow Li's advice, as I noted that many of them bought Daren Lingzhi from the makeshift pharmacy in the back of the hall. By the end of the day, about five hundred people had completed the health survey at the "Say Good-bye to Sniffles" health fair.

Months later Li and I had a discussion about the results and analyses of the survey. He offered his thoughts as follows:

Tired, tired, tired—everyone is complaining about how tired they are. Fatigue is the most popular topic when cosmopolitan city dwellers talk about health. My survey shows that two-thirds of the cosmopolitans are either feeling tired or suffering from chronic fatigue syndrome. This kind of fatigue is different from the type that affects manual laborers and peasants. It's the fatigue of the mind-body. "Mind-body fatigue" . . . refers to fatigue caused by stress, tension, psychological and emotional trauma, and prolonged overuse of the brain. The cause of this fatigue is mostly emotional and psychological, and it commonly affects the brain and the neural system, the cardiovascular system, the hormones, and the immune system. The long-term consequence of the mind-body fatigue is more serious than physical fatigue. I conducted a national survey a couple of years ago and discovered that intellectuals, academics, and white-collar workers under the age of forty have much worse health than factory workers and peasants. They are also much more likely to suffer from depression, chronic pain, and insomnia. They have a life expectancy that is 3.26 years shorter. So, there you have it. Traditional Chinese medicine, which is all about the balancing of body and mind, is the best preventive medicine for the cosmopolitan.

The kind of behavioral medicine that Li refers to in this narrative was first explored by a number of medical scientists and doctors in the United States at the end of the 1960s. Although research articles about mind-body health started appearing in authoritative science and medical journals such as *Nature, Journal of the American Medical Association, New England Journal of Medicine,* and *Lancet* as early as 1975, it is only within the past few years that behavioral medicine became a popular health concept and practice, especially in California's corporate culture (see, e.g., Eisenberg et al. 1993, 1998). Li, in a few words, has captured the gist of this cutting-edge and controversial approach to medicine and health—not only its focus on the mind-body connection but also its clientele, the white-collar middle class.

It is noteworthy that Li's observations of the content and clientele of his new preventive medicine are also mediated by his experience as a "sent-down youth" during the Cultural Revolution, when the party-state sent urban youth en masse to rural China in an effort to develop these areas and also to reeducate urban youth in proletariat virtues. Li worked in a rural factory for years and became familiar with the kind of fatigue resulting from manual labor. Thus he insists that mind-body fatigue is different from what affects manual laborers and peasants, and has "more serious" long-term consequences. Reinterpreting Chinese medical theories about the triangulated, dependent, and transformative relations of qi, *xue* (blood), and *jinye* (bodily fluid)—each of which takes on a more condensed form—Li argues that whereas fatigue caused by manual labor damages *weiqi* (defensive yang qi that guards the body), mind-body fatigue hurts *xue* and *jinye*. Whereas syndromes associated with *weiqi* damage are relatively superficial and easy to treat (for example, the common cold), those associated with problems in *xue* and *jinye* tend to run a prolonged course and are therefore more difficult to completely uproot (for example, high blood pressure, stroke, and insomnia). Thus Li's promotion of mind-body health and medicine—especially his insistence that traditional Chinese medicine is the perfect preventive medicine for the cosmopolitan middle class—is mediated not only by his medical expertise, but also by his experiences and haunting memories of socialist China.

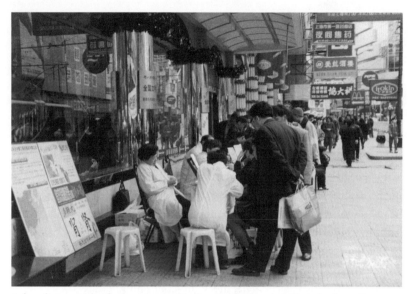

A free clinic outside of a drugstore on Nanjing Road, Shanghai. Photo by the author.

The concept of yajiankang caught on very quickly in urban China, especially through its promotion by practitioners of traditional Chinese medicine. Though yajiankang was still a new medical term in the late 1990s, within a few years it entered the Shanghainese vocabulary of everyday conversation. Today there are journals, websites, workshops, and international conferences on yajiankang. In 2006, a local survey in Shanghai suggested that, among the Shanghainese, only 5 percent were "truly healthy," 20 percent were "truly sick," and the rest fell under the category of yajiankang (Luo 2006). White-collar workers who worked under stressful conditions became the main victims as experts were quick to link the rise of wealth, as well as urban living and working conditions, with the decline of health (*China Daily* 2005; Watts 2004). Indeed, when I googled "亚健康" ("subhealth") on March 7, 2007, a total of 316,000 entries were displayed in less than a second. The market seems promising for the new preventive medicine.

Li's own experimentation with science, medicine, and community building did not stop with the invention of yajiankang. I met with him in September 1999, after he had just returned from La Semaine Chinoise in Paris, where he gave a presentation on traditional Chinese medicine in front of a French audience. Looking sharper than ever in his Parisian fashions, Li told me that his research institute had developed a new formula medicine, an improved, more potent version of Daren Lingzhi. He named it "Act," an English word. Why an English name for a traditional Chinese herbal product? Li explained, "The well-educated young people would know what it means. Besides, 'Act' just sounds exotic."

As noted by Sheldon Pollock and others (2002:1), specifying cosmopolitanism positively and definitely is an uncosmopolitan thing to do. In my view, part of the allure of cosmopolitanism lies precisely in its elusiveness—its resistance to fixation by time or scale. Cosmopolitanism is not the antithesis of local, and it is not an extension of the national. It is not the cultural expression of the global, and neither is it distinctively novel: the international proletariat is but one of the many fading, though unforgotten, cosmopolitan dreams.[11] These old dreams continue to haunt us, mediate new aspirations, and are sometimes recycled in unpredictable ways.[12]

What cosmopolitanism does bring to the fore are the multiple, shifting, and sometimes competing worldly visions mediated by particular kinds of translocal affiliations and entangled in specific terms of differences. In tracing the trajectories and practices of traditional Chinese medicine through different historical periods and across seemingly disparate yet interconnected sites, I suggest that the worlding of traditional Chinese medicine articulates and transfigures, rather than transcends and obliterates, the politics of race and class, knowledge and identity. By conducting ethnographic studies on the ground we may be able to examine and understand world-making projects and processes—such as "globalization"—that have been held up to us in totalizing ways. Instead of trying to conceptually contain or catch up with globalization, we may try catching projects and processes in action.

One of these world-making projects and processes takes us to Africa, where Chinese medicine was worlded in the 1960s and 1970s. In November 2006 China hosted the Beijing Summit and Third Ministerial Conference of Forums on China-Africa Cooperation. As the biggest diplomatic event ever hosted by the People's Republic of China, it was attended by government leaders from forty-eight of the fifty-three countries of Africa. News reports, stories, and images of Africa—as well as the China-Africa relationship—inundated newspapers, websites, and even billboards along the streets of Chinese cities. Among these stories and images the Chinese medical teams—especially the acupuncturists—again took center stage, as reflected by sensational headlines such as "Chinese Acupuncture Cures African Princess," "Ten Years against Malaria in Africa," and "Thousands of Marvelous Chinese Doctors in Africa." Further, the Chinese Ministry of Health claimed that, in addition to the rise in the number of Chinese medical entrepreneurs, there were more than 950 government-sent Chinese medical professionals in over thirty-six African countries, "spreading the love from Chinese people to African people" (Sina.com 2006b).

"Love," however, is far from innocent. Rather than promoting an international proletariat brotherhood, the summit focused on "partnerships" in trade, economic aid for Africa, and cultural exchange. Critics in Europe and North America were quick to argue that China was merely exploiting Africa for its resources and markets—in short, doing the same thing that the British had done a hundred years ago (see, e.g., Kahn 2006; Tisdall 2006; Walsh 2006). These vociferous concerns accentuate the rising anxieties from Europe and North America over China's perceived ascendance in a changing global order. Although such concerns perform a kind of social critique, they are often impeded by a poverty of imagination and of memory. On the one hand, these critiques reproduce a familiar and limited repertoire of tropes—poverty, destitution, and backwardness—that has characterized and shaped colonial and postcolonial Euro-American humanitarian discourses about Africa. On the other hand, they fail to recognize the complexity and historicity of China's engagements with Africa.

China's "return" to Africa, as well as the critical response from Western media and state organizations that ensued, also generated much interest and discussions in academia (see, e.g., Alden 2007; Alden et al. 2008; Lee forthcoming; Sautman and Yan 2007, 2008). These discussions highlight the fact that China's role in Africa cannot be easily categorized as colonizer, partner, or competitor (Alden 2007). While some African workers openly resist the commercial and labor practices of Chinese companies and entrepreneurs in Africa, African states often look to China for a model of sustainable development different from that of the West (Lee forthcoming; Sautman and Yan 2007). Stacey Langwick (2010), for example, argues that the Tanzanian state and some medical practitioners find the reinvention of traditional Chinese medicine a useful model for transforming and scientizing Tanzania's traditional healing practice. Furthermore, even as China emphasizes trade in its current relations with Africa, Chinese policies and activities are distinct from those of Western colonialism and imperialism, especially because of the shared and yet also divergent history and experience of socialism and postsocialism that links China to a number of African countries. As noted by Elisabeth Hsu (2002, 2008), although private clinics and entrepreneurial medicine have come to replace state-sponsored Chinese medical teams, these private Chinese physicians continue to benefit from the reputation of Chinese medical teams during the Mao era.

Thus, even though China's new global economic and political ambitions are articulated through its efforts to "get on track" with Europe and North America, these ambitions and dreams also thrive on rekindling the remembrances of the proletariat world. In an interview with reporters during the China-Africa forums the Chinese foreign minister Li Zhaoxing stated: "In October 1971 it was mainly because of the support from African countries and other friendly nations, that the new China regained its lawful position at the United Nations. When a friend did us a favor, we should remember it forever" (Sina.com 2006b).[13] Without mentioning the name of Mao Zedong, Li quoted Mao's old saying, "In this world, there is no love without a cause [shijieshang meiyou wuyuanwugu de ai]." Whereas the "cause" (*yuangu*) in Mao's original utterance was a reference to impassioned class struggles and alliances, Li's strikingly candid comment was not only an allusion to old patterns of solidarity but also suggestive of what these yuangu—as well as the kinds of worlds they enable—might look like today.

Two

HANDS, HEARTS, AND DREAMS

Marianne was a third-year student at a University of California campus in the San Francisco Bay Area. Having always been interested in biology and chemistry, she became intrigued by the work of Andrew Weil, an M.D. based in Arizona who is now one of the most well-known gurus and entrepreneurs of complementary and alternative medicine (CAM). In her words, "science means an open mind" and therefore she felt that it was perfectly logical for her to pursue a different kind of medical practice. When I first met her in 1999, she was considering enrollment in the American College of Traditional Chinese Medicine (ACTCM) in San Francisco after graduating from the University of California.

However, her decision was not viewed by her family as a good one, and her father, a surgeon at a Bay Area hospital, was adamant in his objection. It was during this tug of war that I was invited to have dinner at the home of Marianne's parents—a dinner at which Marianne's career choice was the obvious source of tension. In an effort to strike up a conversation, Marianne told her father about my research and asked if he had had any contact with traditional Chinese medicine. He replied immediately, "Yes, I know what Chinese medicine is. We have acupuncture at our pain management center now. Of course Chinese medicine is 'complementary' to Western medicine." Just as Marianne and I were beginning to breathe a sigh of relief, he added slyly, "It's always nice to have someone hold your hands."

I was struck by both the perceptiveness of this remark and its undisguised dismissal and contempt of acupuncture. The comment by Marianne's father about hand holding refers to the act of pulse taking in traditional Chinese medicine. Pulse taking is both a trademark diagnostic technique in which many accomplished practitioners take great pride, as well as a source of accusations of vagueness and softness from opponents and even young students of traditional Chinese medicine. "To have someone hold your hands" also alludes to the insistence by many proponents of traditional Chinese medicine that it is a kinder—and in this sense "softer"—medical practice that takes into consideration the "human" in the fullest sense, especially compared to biomedicine. In California, for example, the popularity of traditional Chinese medicine and other CAM practices such as chiropractic and homeopathy largely arose out of—and is sustained by—patients' dissatisfaction with biomedicine's focus on the disease rather than the patient as the primary object of diagnosis and treatment, as well as the exorbitant cost of biomedicine and the oligarchy of health insurance establishments. In his remarks, Marianne's father targeted the ambiguity of the double "softness" of Chinese medicine: he picked out pulse taking so that he could belittle rather than understand it, and he raised an important reason why patients were drawn to Chinese medicine, only to trivialize it.

In this chapter I take seriously what Marianne's father so cleverly highlighted and quickly dismissed. Rather than positing traditional Chinese medicine as the softer counterpart of biomedicine, I take a close look at how entanglements with biomedicine and especially translocal processes of commodification have reconstituted the everyday sociality of Chinese medicine—not only in terms of its stakes and objectives but also in the production of pedagogical and clinical knowledge and expertise. In doing so, I argue that instead of reducing knowledges and ethics to market logic and exchange values, processes of commodification generate new sites where the clinical and pedagogical knowledge and practice of traditional Chinese medicine are creatively and meaningfully reorganized, negotiated, and performed.

During my fieldwork in Shanghai and in the Bay Area, I became accustomed to the sight of red silk banners lining the hallways and treatment rooms of many traditional Chinese clinics and hospitals. As grateful presents from patients and eloquent advertisements for clinics and practitioners, the banners were inscribed with calligraphy that praised the practitioners' skills and kindness. The inscription *renxin renshu*, which means "kind heart and kind skills," was one of the most popular. For their part, practitioners and textbooks of traditional Chinese medicine have emphasized, in theory if not always in practice, the equally important twin concepts of the "virtue of medical practice" (*yide*) and the "skill of medical practice" (*yishu*). Activists and proponents of traditional Chinese medicine often invoke yide and yishu to set traditional Chinese medicine apart, in their view, from the more impersonal and commodified world of biomedicine. For this reason, they are also wary that the participation in mainstream healthcare, which is heavily commodified in both China and the United States, threatens the integrity of Chinese medicine. Yet those who object to traditional Chinese medicine single out its emphasis on yishu and especially yide in order to discredit it for being a soft medicine—namely, more of an art than science, and all about being kind rather than curing diseases.

Ambiguous entanglements with biomedical discourses, practices, and institutions—further complicated by the processes of commodification—are thus at the center of the everyday sociality of traditional Chinese medicine. Rather than creating a level field for the translocal circulation of commodities and values, encounters with biomedicine and entanglements in commodification have created shifting and uneven terrains of power and meaning where yide and yishu of traditional Chinese medicine are put to the test, remolded, and at times caught in life-and-death tussles. In what follows, I discuss and compare the positionalities and predicaments of traditional Chinese medicine vis-à-vis biomedicine and commodification in Shanghai and in the San Francisco Bay Area, while navigating through various institutional and sociohistorical sites. Chinese medicine on both sides of the Pacific has been caught up in the processes of commodification—through its entrance and participation as a form of CAM in mainstream healthcare in San Francisco and through the marketization and privatization of healthcare reform in Shanghai. In San Francisco, Chinese medicine has experienced a change of fortune from being resolutely excluded by biomedicine to being embraced as a more holistic and less costly alternative by patients and, to a lesser extent, by biomedical institutions and professionals. In Shanghai, in contrast, medical professionals including practitioners of traditional Chinese medicine have come to bear the brunt of a healthcare reform that has all but failed. Marketization and privatization have driven patients with limited financial resources further away from Chinese medicine and toward biomedical hospitals and clinics. In their struggles to gain footing in an increasingly narrow professional space, some practitioners refashion themselves into entrepreneurs by opening private practices, promoting new health concepts such as subhealth, and marketing new medicinal products. Some seek their fortunes by immigrating and setting up shop overseas. Some practitioners and students have even abandoned the profession altogether. Those who remain at public hospitals and clinics often not only find themselves pressured to make a profit, but also easy targets of disgruntled patients who take out their resentment against the current state of healthcare on individual doctors, nurses, and hospitals. These resentments are sometimes intensified by the perceived disparity between the traditional ethics and stated goals of Chinese medicine, on the one hand, and the heartlessness of the medical system and practice, on the other. Thus, rather than being overdetermined by the triangulation of traditional Chinese medicine, biomedicine, and commodification, yishu and yide are contested and transformed through sociohistorically specific relations with biomedicine and particular projects of commodification, and take on divergent forms in due process. This chapter aims to explicate the ways in which yishu and yide are negotiated through these relations and projects.

The "American Disease"

In recent decades popular and academic discourses in both China and the United States have become increasingly critical of biomedicine as a lucrative business and an expensive commodity. Fairness and efficiency—or rather the lack thereof—are the focus of these criticisms. In the United States rising healthcare costs and their implications for medical ethics are no longer the subject of criticism only by those actively campaigning against the biomedical establishment, but have now become one of the biggest concerns for the working and middle classes at large. In 2005 healthcare expenditure in the United States reached 2 trillion dollars, or 6,700 dollars per person (Catlin et al. 2006), and it is projected to reach 2.9 trillion dollars in 2009 and 4 trillion dollars by 2015 (Borger et al. 2006). The 2 trillion dollars represented roughly 15 percent of the overall GDP. The problems and reforms of the healthcare system have not only been at the forefront of political debates, especially during presidential elections, but have also drawn heightened media attention. In 2007 the iconoclastic filmmaker Michael Moore's documentary *Sicko* compared the U.S. healthcare system unfavorably to that of Canada, Britain, France, and Cuba. The film, which recorded the second-highest opening day box office for a documentary, struck a chord with the audience by showing that it is not just the medically uninsured but also the insured middle class that have difficulties obtaining affordable and adequate healthcare.

Even though the U.S. healthcare model is far from being the fairest or the most efficient in the world, China has been "very fond" of using the U.S. model as the basis for comparison as it proceeds with its own privatization of healthcare (Wang 2004:42). Today, China's healthcare system, which in the 1960s and 1970s provided rural and urban Chinese with basic care and was lauded by the World Health Organization as an exemplary model for the developing world, now fares worse than the United States in terms of both fairness and efficiency. In urban China, the privatization of healthcare and the withdrawal of state subsidies since the 1990s means that over the period between 1990 and 2004, when personal disposable income more than quintupled, healthcare expenditure increased by almost twenty times (Chinese Academy of Social Science 2007). In 2000 the United States ranked number 54 out of 191 on the WHO scale of "fairness in financial contribution," and China ranked number 188—a great humiliation for a self-styled "socialist" country (Wang 2004:18). This prompted a critical report from the National Reform and Development Commission, a special taskforce established by the Chinese State Council (the executive branch of the central Chinese government). The report publicly lamented that although China's healthcare reform did not exactly copy the American model, it had "contracted the American disease" of inefficiency and unfairness, and that the healthcare reform had been "essentially unsuccessful" (Wang 2005:1). Even as the central government's admission of failure forced the Healthcare Reform Taskforce to search for new paths and plans, for the everyday Chinese the drastic increase in healthcare cost and decrease in performance gave rise to progressively more hostile relations between hospitals and healthcare professionals on the one hand and patients who had been turned into reluctant consumers on the other. Healthcare professionals bear the brunt of the failing healthcare reform: for many Chinese, doctors are no longer "angels in a white coat" (*baiyi tianshi*) but rather personifications of greed and, occasionally, easy targets of intensely felt resentment.

The lack of efficiency and equity in the commodified healthcare poses challenges and opportunities for traditional Chinese medicine. In the

United States, feelings of dissatisfaction with medical establishments—and biomedical institutions in particular—have prompted patients to regard "traditional" healing practices as an alternative that is more holistic, kinder, and often cheaper than biomedicine. In China, where tensions between doctors and patients are at a historical high, traditional Chinese medicine seems to provide a less costly and potentially more benign alternative. In Shanghai in 2006, clinical visits at the four division 3 hospitals of traditional Chinese medicine cost well below the average of 246 yuan per clinic visit among all nineteen division 3 hospitals.[1] A clinic visit cost an average of 203 yuan at Shuguang Hospital, 201 yuan at Longhua Hospital, 161 yuan at Yueyang Hospital, and 158 yuan at the Municipal Hospital of Chinese Medicine (Shanghai Municipal Health Bureau 2007). More tellingly still, whereas inpatient cost averaged 905 yuan per day among division 3 hospitals, the cost was only 512 yuan at Yueyang, 508 yuan at Shuguang, 462 yuan at Longhua, and 376 yuan at the Municipal Hospital of Chinese Medicine. This had to do with the fact that, when choosing hospitals for "serious illnesses" that required inpatient treatments, the overwhelming majority of patients chose biomedical hospitals that in turn charged higher prices. Together, the hospitals of traditional medicine ranked as the four lowest in terms of inpatient costs among all division 3 hospitals.

Ambiguous Commodities

The turn to traditional Chinese medicine, however, does not avoid or resolve the problems of a translocal healthcare landscape dominated by biomedical discourses, institutions, and practices. Anthropologists have observed that, rather than a pure alternative to biomedicine, a "traditional" medical practice is transformed in complex ways when appropriated by the biomedical mainstream. Critical medical anthropology has long questioned biomedicine's almost exclusive focus on the anatomicopathological, the facts of anatomy and pathology that underlie the reification of "disease" as the primary object of medical intervention and leave the patient's illness experience out of medical discourses (see, e.g., Baron 1985; Chavez 2004; Lock 1988; Lock and Scheper-Hughes 1987). Margaret Lock (1990) in her analysis of contemporary practices of Japanese herbal medicine, which has deep roots in Chinese herbal medicine, points to the phenomena of rationalization and fragmentation as well as to those of commodification and medicalization.

"Rationalization" refers to the process by which the conceptual under-pinnings of traditional healing practices are translated and reinterpreted through the existing conceptual repertoire of biomedicine and biological science. Rationalization often fails to embrace or legitimize elements of medical practices that cannot be easily explained within the scope of bio-medicine and thus tends to simply write off incongruence and contradic-tion—which results in the fragmentation of traditional medical practices. For example, laboratory research on "active ingredients" in various herbal medicines has targeted finding chemical compounds that would suppress if not cure specific diseases. Successful researches in active ingredients (i.e., double-blind and replicable experiments in which active and therapeuti-cally effective chemicals are successfully isolated and tested) lend limited legitimacy to herbal medicines. In the meantime, the search for active in-gredients often discards medical philosophies and principles that are in-congruent with biomedicine—even though these philosophies and prin-ciples serve as the basis for the use of herbs in traditional medicines. As one practitioner of traditional Chinese medicine in San Francisco stated suc-cinctly in a conversation with me, the approach of Chinese herbal medicine is "constructive" in the sense that, through carefully balanced herbal pre-scriptions, it aims to adjust the overall bodily constitutions of the patient as he or she goes through various stages over the course of an illness. In contrast, biomedicine is "destructive" in the sense that it relies on the iden-tification of diseases and, more precisely, pathogens (e.g., germs or can-cer cells) that then must be destroyed. The search for "active ingredients," while in keeping with biomedicine's destructive approach to disease, does not take into consideration how clinical practices of traditional Chinese medicine conceptualize the human in fluid, open-ended, and transforma-tive ways.

Furthermore, accurate quantification and standardized prescription, though important in biomedicine and in bioscientific research on tradi-tional herbal medicines, are not essential to the practice of Chinese medi-cine. An herbal prescription in Chinese medicine for one course of treat-ment usually consists of about sixteen different kinds of herbs, animal products, and minerals.[2] The prescription is to be taken over a period of one or two weeks, with the exact number of days or doses depending on how fast the syndrome is expected to change and, in some difficult cases, how confident the practitioner is about their handling of the illness and patient.[3] At Shuguang Hospital, which like all comprehensive hospitals in urban China has its own pharmacy, the patient takes the herbalist's or acupuncturist's prescription to the herbal pharmacy where it is dispensed. The pharmacy stores herbs in the small drawers of large wall-to-wall wooden medicinal cabinets, where they are classified according to their medicinal properties.[4] After reviewing the prescription, the pharmacist weighs out the herbs on a handheld balance called a *cheng* before mixing and wrapping up the ingredients in individual paper packages, each of which contains a single dosage of the prescribed mixture of herbs.[5] Shuguang Hospital and all other hospitals of Chinese medicine in Shanghai also offer services in preparing herbal soups for patients who do not have the time or patience to spend hours cooking an herbal concoction. In the hospitals the herbs are cooked in industrial-sized pots, and the liquid is extracted and filtered before being vacuum sealed in individual plastic packages. Patients simply refrigerate these packages and heat them up before use.[6]

Experienced pharmacists are also known for their extensive knowledge of herbal medicine, and their opinions are respected by herbal doctors. While apprenticing at Shuguang Hospital, I noticed occasional incidences in which pharmacists would refuse to fill a prescription that they considered erroneous or inappropriate. Most of these rejected prescriptions were written by junior and inexperienced practitioners. On one occasion, however, a pharmacist rejected a prescription that contained thirty grams of *jiegeng*, or radix platycodi. Jiegeng is a commonly used herb in the treatment of wind-heat type colds (*fengre ganmao*). But because of its mild toxicity, which could cause vomiting, the dose of jiegeng usually does not exceed ten grams. A senior practitioner at Shuguang Hospital, however, had made a name for himself by using large doses of jiegeng—so much so that he was nicknamed Wang Jiegeng. Like many senior practitioners, over his career Wang had become extremely skillful in creatively using a particular herb in ways that exceeded the conventions of textbooks or what was taught by his teachers. It later turned out that the rejected prescription was originally written by Wang Jiegeng, but the apprentice who copied it for the pharmacy signed the prescription in his own name by mistake. Upon hearing who the true author of the prescription was, the pharmacist duly dispensed the herbs.

The administration of herbs is thus not only determined by the syndromes being treated but also is contingent upon the clinical expertise, experience, and preference of individual practitioners.[7] The standardized uses of herbs are not always considered pivotal in Chinese herbal medicine, and herbs are not weighed out meticulously. More importantly, accomplished practitioners such as Wang Jiegeng identify themselves with and distinguish themselves through expertise in using certain uncommon herbs, or in prescribing herbs in unusual quantities or in unexpected combinations. Dr. Ma Zhongjie, another herbalist at Shuguang Hospital, is known for his unconventional usage of *yanhusuo* (rhyzoma corydalis or fumewort), which is used to promote the circulation of blood (*huoxue*) and is rarely included in prescriptions for colds. Dr. Ma, however, makes yanhusuo his trademark herb by including it in his prescriptions for a wide variety of illnesses and especially common colds. Still another herbalist, Dr. Gu Naiqiang, is an expert in the paired use of *xianmao* (rhyzoma curculiginis) and *xianlingpi* (epimedium or barrenwort) in his prescriptions for patients recovering from breast cancer surgeries, in spite of the fact that these are yang-strengthening herbs usually used for male impotence. The practice of developing trademark herbs among practitioners of traditional Chinese medicine underscores a kind of creative and personal knowledge production that resists standardization and cannot be reflected in the search for active ingredients.

It is noteworthy that herbs containing "active ingredients" are often mass produced and marketed to enrich the repertoire of biomedicine in treating an increasing number of diseases—a process that Lock calls the "commodification" and "medicalization" of traditional medicines. She argues that once a traditional practice becomes part of the institutionalized medicine, it could be transformed so that "its values and objectives become reconciled with those of the dominant social order in question" (1990:45). She notes that, in Japan, herbal medicine has been enlisted to treat new "diseases" such as pollution-related respiratory illnesses and stress-related syndromes. Lock argues that medicalization "serves to deflect attention away from the social level and to transform the problem into an individual one for which the patient is held responsible" (45). Rather than located in the social realm, the cause and treatment of these new diseases becomes medical.

Lock's analysis of medicalization and commodification helps illuminate the transformations of Chinese medicine today. For example, the ubiquity of ginseng and other Chinese herbs in food supplements, soft drinks, and cosmetic products in both Shanghai and California speaks all too eloquently for the commodification of traditional Chinese medicine. Furthermore, as noted in chapter 1, businesses and corporations in California now enlist acupuncture and other CAM practices to treat job-related syndromes such as carpal tunnel and a wide range of stress-related problems; at the same time, enterprising practitioners in Shanghai have popularized the concept of yajiankang to reframe the ills of urban lifestyle in terms of a new medical condition which in turn requires medical intervention. It is undeniable that the processes of medicalization and commodification are at play here.

But do these processes, together with rationalization and fragmentation, tell us everything about what happens to traditional medicines when they encounter biomedical mainstreams? Although the focus on rationalization, fragmentation, medicalization, and commodification provides a powerful look at the asymmetries of traditional medicines and biomedicine, it does not completely capture the complex socialities that emerge from the encounters and entanglements between traditional Chinese medicine and biomedicine. First, the analysis of rationalization and fragmentation lends itself to a reading of traditional medicines as victim and biomedicine as villain. It is useful as a critique of the power dynamics that structure biomedicine and traditional medicines, but does not help us see the ways in which practitioners and institutions of traditional Chinese medicine may negotiate new forms of knowledge and redefine areas of expertise by working *in relation with* biomedical discourses, practices, and institutions. Furthermore, I suggest that although medicalization and commodification radically reshape the knowledge and ethics of traditional medicines, they may not entirely flatten the meaningful practices of yishu and yide in traditional Chinese medicine and reduce Chinese medicine to an accomplice of biomedicine. Rather, processes of rationalization, fragmentation, medicalization, and commodification may provide new and contingent terrains upon which formerly impossible dreams—and indeed nightmares—come to realization.

Incidentally, my own entry into traditional Chinese medicine began in a biology laboratory where as a college student in Claremont, California, I participated in testing the effects of the solutions of a number of Chinese herbs on small-cell lung cancer cell cultures. I became intrigued, first and foremost, by the complex ways in which science is produced in the wet lab rather than presented in standardized textbooks. Doing science was at once messy and creative, liberating and daunting—and always interpretive. At the same time, I became acutely aware of and puzzled by both the technical advantages and conceptual limitations of laboratory research on Chinese medicine. Most importantly, perhaps, I was struck by the urgency and earnestness—mingled with anticipation for research breakthroughs and achievements—felt among the participants of this laboratory research project in their pursuit of a solution or even a cure for small-cell lung cancer. It would not be an exaggeration to say that my experience in the lab was the beginning of my own anthropological inquiries into traditional Chinese medicine and my long-term engagement with the social and cultural studies of how science and knowledge are actually produced.

I would like to think, then, that entanglements with biomedicine and processes of commodification are more complex and ambiguous than the decline and demise of the authentic knowledge and ethical integrity of traditional Chinese medicine. Whereas the treatment philosophy of traditional Chinese medicine might be considered "constructive" and that of biomedicine "destructive," I suggest that the ongoing transformations of traditional Chinese medicine are destructive to an extent, and yet constructive in the sense that they produce new forms of sociality that engender new areas of expertise and new objectives. Several anthropologists have already observed the ways in which traditional Chinese medicine is reconstructed, rather than simply appropriated and undermined, through commodification and marketization. Judith Farquhar (1995) in her study of rural, individual entrepreneurial (*getihu*) practitioners of traditional Chinese medicine noted that, at the beginning of the 1990s, small-scale private entrepreneurial practitioners had already begun to quietly replace socialist, collectivist heroes such as Lei Feng. They did so by cultivating a personal "aura" around their clinical practices, which in turn became an attraction for their patients. Participation in marketization thus has personalized rather than alienated the practice of Chinese medicine. The commodification of traditional Chinese medicine has also taken place in what was once the "proletariat world." Elisabeth Hsu (2002) observed that in Tanzania both Chinese biomedical healthcare and traditional Chinese medicine are now increasingly provided by small-scale entrepreneurial Chinese practitioners. Hsu points out that it is precisely the entrepreneurial setup of this brand of Chinese medicine that distinguishes it from bureaucratic "hospital medicine," as well as traditional Tanzanian healing practices and gives it a mass appeal that allows it to flourish.

Both Farquhar and Hsu point to the ways in which traditional Chinese medicine is made through, rather than in spite of, processes of commodification and practices of entrepreneurship—as well as through, in Hsu's case in particular, fraught relations with various forms of biomedicine and other traditional medicines. Building on their discussions, and with a focus on the enmeshment of knowledge and ethics through discourses of renxin renshu, I explore the ways in which shifting forms of traditional Chinese medicine are produced and contested, rather than invariably compromised, through discourses and practices of rationalization and commodification. The processes of rationalization and commodification are at the heart of the everyday practice of Chinese medicine by challenging it, threatening it, and at the same time enabling it to emerge in new forms.

In what follows, I discuss the entwined processes of rationalization and commodification through two concepts: "heart" (*xin*) and "dream" (*mengxiang*). These two words came up repeatedly during my fieldwork when practitioners, teachers, and students spoke of their personal choices of, involvements with, and aspirations for traditional Chinese medicine. I understand the discourses of heart in four ways: first, heart as a discreet organ understood by the bioscientific, anatomical view of the body; second, heart in traditional Chinese medical theory as a part of a symbolic-functional visceral system that is often conflated with but does not correspond to the biomedical heart (Kaptchuk 2000; Scheid 2002); three, the binary notion of heart, which is the domain of the emotional, the irrational, and the occult opposed to "mind"; and, fourth, commonsense understandings in both China and the United States of heart that associate it with kindness, softness, and morality. I suggest that all four concepts of the heart are at play, sometimes in tandem and sometimes in conflict, in shaping yide and yishu today.

Although understanding "heart" differently, many practitioners and students of traditional Chinese medicine speak the common language of "dream" when looking back at the history of Chinese medicine and also looking forward. These dreams, however, vary greatly. Practitioners in California have long dreamed for a legitimate status in mainstream healthcare and have strived for that dream. In the meantime those in China, where traditional Chinese medicine has been a part of institutionalized healthcare since the 1950s, continue to struggle for equity with biomedicine—now in an increasingly commodified environment. Instead of reframing and reducing the expertise and ethics of Chinese medicine to market values, marketization and commodification pose both challenges and opportunities for particular personal and professional dreams of practitioners, teachers, and students. Whereas some cherished dreams are fulfilled after long periods of encounters and entanglements with biomedicine, other dreams turn into nightmares.

Unsettled Hearts

Pulse taking (*damai*) is one of the four basic diagnostic techniques of Chinese medicine. The other techniques are *wang*, or "look," which includes observing the patient's complexion, hair, and fingernails and the color, shape, texture, and coating of the tongue; *wen*, a Chinese character that means both "hearing" (to know if there is any shortness of breath or moans) and "smelling" (of urine and feces); and *wen*, pronounced in the fourth tone,[8] which means "ask" and refers to the process of querying the patient.

During my time at various clinics in Shanghai and the Bay Area, I noticed that practitioners asked questions ranging from the specifics of a clinical case (e.g., particular manifestations of a cold—whether there is phlegm or cough, and at what time of the day the cough is most severe) to routine questions such as the patient's appetite and sleeping patterns. In Shanghai older patients might go to a practitioner, sit down, and hold out their wrists without saying a word. This gesture at once demonstrates the patient's familiarity with and understanding of the diagnostic procedure and is often seen by the practitioner as a "test" that requires the practitioner to ask carefully selected questions. As one senior practitioner told his students and apprentices: "When a patient comes in without saying a word, you have to figure out ways to have the patient open his mouth. This skill is not something you learn from the books. You have to ask 'How long have you been ill' because this is not something you can tell from feeling the pulse. If they reply 'five months' then you have to ask 'What was it like before the five months? How does it feel at the end of the five months?' Now you have struck up a conversation. In the end you don't have to ask any questions because the patient will tell you everything on his own." Accomplished senior practitioners are almost invariably masterful at asking questions that animate long responses and thereby a detailed diagnosis without arousing the patient's suspicion of their clinical competence.

Among the four diagnostic techniques, pulse taking is widely considered to be the most important one. In clinics in Shanghai when I asked to take pictures of a practitioner and the patient, the patient often automatically held out the wrist, placed it on the desk facing up, and invited the practitioner to put their fingers on it in the pose of pulse taking—just so that I could take a picture of traditional Chinese medicine in action. During pulse taking the practitioner places his or her forefinger, middle finger, and right finger pressed together on the inside of the patient's wrist, with the forefinger pressed against the bottom of the patient's first metacarpal (thumb). The position on the patient's wrist underneath the practitioner's forefinger is called *cun*, the middle finger *guan*, and the ring finger *chi*. The cun, guan, and chi positions on the left wrist correspond to the visceral systems of heart and small intestine, liver and gall bladder, and kidney, and on the right correspond to lung and large intestine, spleen and stomach, and kidney and bladder.[9] Taken together, the six pulse positions are important indicators of the state of the five *zang* and six *fu* visceral systems.

The main components of the *zangfu* systems are, on the one hand, the five zang systems of heart, lung, spleen, liver, and kidney. They are paired with six fu systems: stomach, small intestine, large intestine, bladder, gall bladder, and *sanjiao*, an anatomically unlocatable system sometimes translated as "triple warmer." In these paired relations, the zang systems are yin symbols of which the main function is to store and nourish, whereas the fu systems are yang, or transformative symbols. It bears mentioning that the yinyang relations noted here are strictly relational in the sense that they are only meaningful when defined against specific counterparts, and their gendered properties can morph depending on specific relational contexts. For example, the heart is described as a yin system in relation to its counterpart the small intestine. However, yin is a relational state of being rather than a fixed property; that is, rather than being a fixed "yin" system, the heart itself is divided into the *yin* of the heart (*xinyin*) and the yang of the heart (*xinyang*).[10]

The zangfu visceral systems are an important representation of how the human body and human constitution are understood in Chinese medicine. In spite of their names (which are the result of translations of biomedical anatomical terms *into* Chinese), "heart," "spleen," "kidney," and so on are not "real" organs in that they do not correspond to anatomical parts of the body. The erroneous assumption that the zangfu systems are an archaic, less accurate version of modern anatomy, however, is prevalent among biomedical professionals, the general public, and even young students of traditional Chinese medicine, and it has been appropriated to argue that Chinese medicine is more vague and less scientific than biomedicine. Today, some practitioners of traditional Chinese medicine propose that the zangfu systems are best understood as symbolic and functional rather than ana-tomicopathological and flesh-and-blood.[11]

Even as practitioners and educators of traditional Chinese medicine struggle to redefine the zangfu system in relation to biomedical anatomy, some young students find it simply too elusive to grasp. Some consider it more difficult than the *jingluo* system—the system of meridians through which qi flows. Students in both Shanghai and San Francisco told me that it is relatively easy for them to envision the jingluo system, which has no exact counterpart in biomedicine. They do so through metaphors of roads, rail-ways, or the nervous system (which they understand is different from the jingluo system). Due to its conflation with anatomical parts in both medical and popular discourses, however, the zangfu system sometimes prove more challenging for young students, especially those trained in high schools in China. Thus, translated comparability—rather than incomparability—obstructs instead of facilitates understanding and raises doubts about Chi-nese medicine rather than clarifies it.

Shi Huizhong was a first-year student at the Shanghai University of Tra-ditional Chinese Medicine (SUTCM) when I first met him in a class called "Basic Theories in Traditional Chinese Medicine," an introductory course required of all SUTCM students. We often sat near each other in the back of the classroom. As a fledgling ethnographer I preferred the back of the room, where I was involved in the action but not quite at the center of it. Shi sat in the back of the classroom for quite different reasons. During breaks he would discuss the lectures with me, often in a quiet voice and especially when his commentaries were critical of the lectures—and they often were. Shi was by no means a "bad student." He usually arrived before me, and I often found him, along with quite a few other students, diligently reading an English textbook until the class started. Several students told me that they considered English one of the most important skills to master during their training at SUTCM. As Shi put it, "English will open many doors—we have a lot of alumni who went to America to practice acupuncture."

Similar to the cases of some of his classmates, SUTCM was not the col-lege Shi dreamed of. Shi was born in Shanghai, and although his grandfa-ther was an herbalist Shi had wanted to go to a medical school—a biomedi-cal one. He was, however, worried that he would not score high enough on the college entrance examination to qualify for either Shanghai Medi-cal University or Shanghai No. 2 Medical University, the two biomedical universities in Shanghai. So he put down SUTCM as his first choice of medical college and was accepted in the first round. In an effort to make sense of his career, he stated: "Biomedicine would have been the choice of my *mind*. Chinese medicine is the choice of my *heart*."

Shi was not alone in his career choice. To be sure, a considerable number of students who enter SUTCM are genuinely interested in traditional Chinese medicine. Others choose SUTCM for various reasons including, for example, the fact that they believe that traditional Chinese medicine is an appropriate profession for female students because it requires the practitioner to be meticulous, patient, and affectionate (for more on the gendering of traditional Chinese medicine, see chapter 5). However, a number of students enter SUTCM because Shanghai Medical University and Shanghai No. 2 University are out of their reach. As in any other part of China, a student in Shanghai is usually required to take the college entrance examination, the score of which is used to decide which university, college, or professional school they will enter if they meet the cutoff line.[12] However, unlike other parts of China, which use the standardized national examinations, Shanghai prepares and administers its own exams. Before taking the exams, which last several days, each student is requested to fill out an application form for their desired institutions and rank their preferences.[13] At the entrance exams, a high school student is always tested in the disciplines of Chinese, English, and mathematics. Depending on their specialization (the choice of which has been made earlier), the student is also examined in one of the following disciplines: history, geography, or politics if they have chosen disciplines of literature (*wenke*), which are comparable to the humanities and social sciences; and physics, chemistry, or biology if they have chosen disciplines of rationality (*like*), which are comparable to the natural sciences.

Medical schools take rationality (*like*) students only, with the exception of SUTCM which allocates a very small quota to literature (*wenke*) students under the assumption that they will have an advantage in studying and specializing in ancient medical texts. Because relative to SUTCM both Shanghai Medical University and Shanghai No. 2 Medical University set higher cutoff scores, SUTCM often gets students who either fail to enter the two biomedical universities or, like Shi, those who make SUTCM their first choice to play it safe.[14] Within SUTCM, the admission cutoff score for the Department of Chinese Medicine (*zhongyi xi*) is higher than that of the Department of Acupuncture (*zhenjiu xi*), which in turn is higher than that of the Department of Herbal Pharmacology (*zhongyao xi*)—the graduates of which are mostly likely to work as herbal pharmacists.[15]

One result of the hierarchy enforced by the entrance exams among the medical universities is that SUTCM often receives students trained in physics, chemistry, and biology who find the conceptual underpinnings of traditional Chinese medicine to be antithetic to the views they spent at least six years learning and internalizing in high school. I often heard complaints from first- and second-year students that Chinese medicine is too vague, soft, and "difficult to explain" (*shuobuqing*); that the courses are repetitive; and that the biomedical training offered by SUTCM as part of their curriculum is not up to the standards of the biomedical universities.

For their part, the faculty and clinicians who instruct interns are confident that the students at SUTCM receive ample training in biomedical concepts and techniques that are in no way inferior to those offered by the two biomedical universities. They are also often dissatisfied with the attitude and competence of their younger students, and they are troubled by what they see as a lack of commitment, interest, and intellectual vigor from students. For these teachers, the four-year college training is also a process of the transformation and conversion of their students, the result of which is by no means guaranteed.

Shi is certainly not the only student who invokes the division between heart and mind to discuss his view of and career in traditional Chinese medicine. It is a sentiment echoed by many students of traditional Chinese medicine in Shanghai. Ironically, the opposition of emotion to rationality, which is "common sense" among students, is grounded in the Cartesian dualism that has long been critiqued as the basis for biomedicine's reification of disease and alienation of lived experience (Kleinman 1995; Lock and Scheper-Hughes 1987). Yet many of these young hearts remain unsettled— not the anatomical heart in biomedicine or the symbolic-functional heart in traditional Chinese medicine, but the philosophical heart of Cartesian dualism that has made the anatomical heart real and the heart of the zangfu system elusive. Shi himself never became a practitioner of traditional Chinese medicine. After graduation, he began working as a sales representative for the China branch of a large American pharmaceutical company. He was fortunate in finding a lucrative job: graduates from SUTCM are sometimes rejected by multinational companies on the grounds that those trained in traditional Chinese medicine have an archaic mind that is out of sync with the tempo of the hectic modern world.

California Dreams

One of Shi Huizhong's dreams was to move to California and become a successful acupuncturist. Although some students in Shanghai are trying to leave the profession of traditional Chinese medicine (or stay in it only reluctantly), in California the colleges and academies of Chinese medicine have been enjoying surging popularities for the last two decades.

In California and in the United States more broadly, acupuncture and Chinese herbal medicine have emerged as part of the diverse set of therapeutic practices institutionalized in the form of CAM. The scope of CAM has been shifting over the years. In 1998 David Eisenberg and his colleagues conducted a telephone survey on the use of alternative medicine. Among the sixteen therapies covered by the survey were such diverse methods as acupuncture, acupressure, chiropractic therapy, homeopathy, ayurveda, biofeedback, guided imagery, relaxation techniques, high-dose vitamin therapy, and prayer. As a follow-up study of the original survey conducted in 1993, the 1998 study involved 2,055 adults in various parts of the United States. The results of the survey note an increase in the number of medical conditions for which alternative medicines are used, with back trouble, allergies, arthritis, and digestive issues listed as some of the main problems. The survey results also show that between 1990 and 1997 visits to practitioners of alternative medicine increased by 47 percent from 427 million to 629 million, and expenditures increased by 45 percent to 21.2 billion, with 12.2 billion out-of-pocket expenses.

The steadily rising popularity of CAM belies the highly difficult route toward the legalization and mainstreaming of acupuncture in the United States, including California. Known by many for its counterculture reputation, California saw the popular support for alternative and spiritual healing practices gather force in the 1960s. Following the normalization of the Sino-U.S. relationship in 1979, grassroots movements in California were boosted by interest on the part of research scientists and biomedical professionals as well as the general public. Some of the most persevering activists, however, were practitioners and patients from diverse backgrounds. Today, by writing various memoirs and histories older practitioners of traditional Chinese medicine still work together as well as compete with each other in reconstructing the history of their struggles (see chapter 1).

Even though these memoirs and histories differ in their accounts of some of the specific events and the important contributors to the legalization of acupuncture, most of them agree that the arrest and trial of Miriam Lee in 1974 was a key event that added momentum to tip the balance in their struggles. Lee was a well-known acupuncturist who had a small clinic in Palo Alto in the 1970s. She was trained as a nurse and a midwife in mainland China before becoming an acupuncturist. A devout Christian, she immigrated to Singapore in 1949 and then later to California. She firmly believed that a kind and effective medical practice such as acupuncture should be made available to anyone who would like to try it. As a result her clinic in Palo Alto became wildly popular, and, according to several of my correspondents, it aroused the jealousy of the wife of a biomedical physician whose nearby clinic was apparently losing business to Lee. Lee's practice was reported to the police, presumably by the physician's wife, and Lee was arrested at her clinic in the early morning of April 16, 1974, one day after Governor Ronald Reagan vetoed a bill that would have legalized acupuncture in California.[16] Lee's subsequent trial in Sacramento galvanized the efforts to legalize acupuncture in California: her patients (some on the arms of their relatives) went to Sacramento to testify to the effectiveness of her medical practice, and local politicians and attorneys were mobilized in her support (many of whom went on to work on legislatures on acupuncture). As a result acupuncture gained more publicity than ever, and Lee was eventually found not to be guilty and her court record was stricken. At the time of my fieldwork in 1998 her Palo Alto clinic was still operating.

Lee's case was one of the first victories toward the legalization of acupuncture in California. The alleged role of the biomedical physician and his wife—as well as the unintended consequences of their action—suggests that commodification was an integral part of this story. Traditional Chinese medicine was seen not only as a different or subversive medical practice but also as an infringement on biomedicine's monopoly of the market. Relations between communities of traditional Chinese medicine and biomedical professionals were complicated and even contentious. Many older practitioners recalled difficulties with biomedical professionals. Liu Hanchao, an herbalist who treated many cancer patients, said that she used to receive calls from callers claiming to be from the American Cancer Association, asking her to "leave our business alone."

The increase in popular demand for acupuncture and Chinese herbal medicine, however, has changed the relation between the communities of traditional Chinese medicine and the biomedical establishments. First, many of the students of traditional Chinese medicine have been patients of acupuncturists and herbalists. In my interviews with students at ACTCM, many told me that their experiences as patients of traditional Chinese medicine had contributed to their decision in pursuing a career in this medical practice. Some of them turned to traditional Chinese medicine for illnesses where biomedicine is ineffective or less effective (see chapter 3). In addition, they noted that they were "turned off" by the sterile attitude, exorbitant cost, and sometimes perceived incompetence of biomedical doctors.

Biomedical institutions and practitioners have, in the words of many practitioners, "turned around." Major Bay Area hospitals and HMOs such as the Chinese Hospital, St. Luke's Hospital, Kaiser Permanente, and the University of California are eager to include acupuncturists in their hospitals and clinics. Major health insurance companies now offer coverage in acupuncture and other kinds of CAM such as chiropractic. Many practitioners of traditional Chinese medicine are bemused if not troubled by the turnaround of the biomedical mainstream. It is not exactly a dream come true. Although many celebrate the newly found status of legitimacy, they also worry about the appropriation by biomedical mainstream and commercial interests. As one acupuncturist and longtime activist put it, "It is a love-hate relation. How can we push acupuncture into the mainstream without entering and competing in the market?"

Redefining Expertise

Whereas in California the processes of commodification and encounters with biomedicine first barred traditional Chinese medicine from the medical mainstream and then propelled it by appropriation and negotiation, practitioners in Shanghai face different challenges—notably those posed by the rapid privatization and marketization of healthcare since the early 1990s.

Beginning in the early 1990s, major hospitals in Shanghai—Shuguang Hospital, Yueyang Hospital, and Longhua Hospital, among others, began competing with each other to invite famous senior doctors of Chinese medicine (*minglao zhongyi*) to join their newly founded "minglao zhongyi expert clinics." Traditional Chinese herbal drugstores such as Caitongde Tang and Tonghanchun Tang also revived the old practice of "sitting in the drugstore" (*zuotang*) by inviting famous doctors to spend a few mornings or afternoons a week treating customers at drugstores.[17] The profit from these events is divided between the practitioners and the hospitals or drugstores.

For example, if a visit to an expert clinic costs 50 yuan (much higher than a regular clinic visit), the hospital would take 60 percent and the practitioner 40 percent. For the practitioners of traditional Chinese medicine, expert clinics and zuotang present opportunities for extra income in addition to their regular salaries. For hospitals and drugstores, an expert-packed clinic not only draws patients and enhances their reputations but also means that they could receive part of the profit without having to pay additional salary to these experts.

Practitioners of traditional Chinese medicine are self-conscious about their participation in the world of commodified and privatized healthcare. Many angle for a spot at a well-paid expert clinic or drugstore. As a minglao zhongyi put it, "It's the economy of commodity now [shangping jingji]. Hospitals have to compete with each other and so do doctors—we all need patients. Doctors have also become commodities themselves."

Yet these famous doctors are more than mere commodities; indeed, they themselves are entrepreneurs. Dr. Hu Erxiong is such as example. I studied with Dr. Hu at an expert clinic where he worked half a day each week. Hu was born in 1940, and his grandfather, father, paternal uncle, and brothers and sisters were all practitioners of traditional Chinese medicine. Hu had inherited the family tradition in practicing the "external medicine of traditional Chinese medicine" (zhongyi waike; where "wai" means "external" and "ke" means "division" or "discipline"). Traditionally zhongyi waike referred, literally, to the treatment of illnesses on or near the surface of the body, as well as the external treatment of some internal illnesses. Today, however, zhongyi waike is perhaps one of the most ambiguous and misunderstood of the branches of traditional Chinese medicine—in part because waike is also the Chinese term for "surgery," which is often seen as a foreign biomedical import. To be sure, there is a history of surgery in China, most notably in the work of the physician Hua Tuo (c. AD 145–208) who was known for his skills in acupuncture, anesthesia, and minor surgeries. In the nineteenth century eye surgery was also quite common in China.[18] These surgeries, which involved working on the "surface" of the physical body compared to internal herbal medicine that aimed at regulating qi, fell conveniently under the umbrella "zhongyi waike." Unfortunately for zhongyi waike, however, today most of the lay public—as well as some healthcare professionals and academics—ignore the fact that "zhongyi waike" and "waike" came from different origins, and instead simply see zhongyi waike as a premodern and inferior variation of modern surgery.

Hu, however, is unfazed by the predicament of zhongyi waike. While his grandfather specialized in the treatment of skin lesions in general and warts in particular, his father developed and extended the family tradition into the herbal treatment of breast cancer and breast fibroids. Hu's clinical practice builds on his father's innovations. In my observation, Hu's patients at the expert clinic were mostly patients with skin problems, or those who were undergoing or recovering from biomedical treatments of breast cancer and fibroids. I was intrigued by Hu's specialization in skin and breast conditions, which I first thought was an odd combination. But Hu explained to me that in traditional Chinese medicine both malignant and benign tumors are called *yan* ("rock" or "hard formation"), and they are caused by *yu*—a process of stagnation and sedimentation. In that sense, warts and fibroids could be considered similar syndromes (*zheng*) and thus treated with the same treatment principle: soften the hard and dissolve the phlegm (*ruanjian huatan*). In practice, he often included softening (*ruanjian*) herbs, such as *muli* (the shell of oyster), *shancigu* (pseudobulbus cremastrae seu pleiones), *haizao* (seaweed), and *kunbu* (thallus laminarae) in his prescription for patients with warts and fibroids. He also often added *banzhilian* (scutellariae barbatae) and *baihuasheshecao* (hedyotis diffusae), popular herbs for cancer treatment by Chinese medicine today, when treating patients suffering or recovering from cancer.

Hu is immensely popular among his patients and nurses, not only because of the effectiveness of his treatment but also because of his yide. He is an amicable man who in everyday practice always tries to find ways to lower medical costs for his patients. On one occasion, a regular patient of Hu's had an argument with one of the nurses over the payment of clinic visit fees. The patient insisted that she had already paid the 50 yuan fee whereas the nurse argued that exactly 50 yuan was missing from her cash register. The patient went into Hu's treatment room still fuming, with the vociferous nurse at her heels. After hearing the story from both sides, Hu simply stepped in and paid the 50 yuan himself. Everybody was pleased. After the patient had left, Hu said to me, "*heqishengcai*," an old saying that means "kindness brings wealth."

In redefining and expanding his areas of expertise as well as fostering the attitude of kindness in medical practice, Hu is one of the entrepreneurial-minded practitioners in Shanghai who have prospered in the marketization of traditional Chinese medicine. He is not without competitors, however. Dr. Wang Shoude, another minglao zhongyi who specializes in *fuke*, or women's illness,[19] was troubled by the ways in which Hu had gained a foothold in the treatment of breast cancer. Dr. Wang, who works at the same expert clinic as Dr. Hu but on different days, considers breast cancer a fuke problem that has been "snatched" by zhongyi waike. In his own practice Dr. Wang often prescribed herbs commonly used in fuke, especially herbs used in the regulation of blood for patients with breast, ovarian, or cervical cancers. His treatment tended to focus on facilitating blood circulation, as Chinese medicine considers many of women's illnesses to be blood-related syndromes. And, like Dr. Hu, Dr. Wang had his own group of faithful patients.

Both Drs. Hu and Wang are senior practitioners who have skillfully and successfully renegotiated their areas of expertise and professional ethics at a time of drastic transformations in Shanghai's healthcare profession. Their successes are shaped by the power-laden relations between biomedicine and Chinese medicine, the commodification of healthcare, and heightened tensions between doctors and patients as well as among doctors themselves. As the knowledges and practices of Chinese medicine become commodified, both Hu and Wang struggle to hold onto a sense of professional identity that at once allows them to rethink and redefine their everyday clinical practice and to thrive successfully in privatized medicine. The commodification of Chinese medicine has thus not simply reduced its knowledge and practices to mere commodities with market values but rather has opened up new sites where renxin renshu is refigured.

Whereas some practitioners participate in expert clinics and practice zuotang at drugstores, others venture even further by setting up their own enterprises. Li Fengyi, one of the first practitioners of traditional Chinese medicine in Shanghai to have opened his own clinic, tries to grapple with the apparent paradox of Chinese medicine as renxin renshu in a marketized healthcare system. He insists that in order for traditional Chinese medicine to survive, it desperately needs to explore new "living space." As he states: "It's all about positioning (dingwei). Chinese medicine has to compete for equal status with biomedicine. Not only in research, but also in the market. I know that in the United States Chinese medicine is considered part of complementary and alternative medicine. Well, that's not going to work in the long run: you are setting limits for yourself by being on equal footing with chiropractors. How far is that going to get you?"

Li has many critics at the university. And he points out to me, defiantly, that he often gets nasty notes from students during and after lectures: "The old timers and their obsolete ideas about Chinese medicine are not go-ing away! No, no, the story does not end with their retirement. They have trained many students—young, passionate students—who call me a traitor. No, the problem is not going away." But perhaps the most ardent critic is Li himself. When I saw him in fall 2003 he was, in spite of his market success, more vocal than ever in speaking up against what he called "the commodi-fication of traditional Chinese medicine." He argued that he was different from other business people because he got into business to "fulfill" a dream (yuanmeng). He noted, "I had been campaigning for Chinese medicine for many years: at conferences, in books and journals, in the classroom. But nobody was paying attention. I have my own thoughts. I am not doing what I do just for money. And now at least I feel like I've accomplished something."

For Drs. Li, Hu, and Wang, as well as many other entrepreneurial-minded practitioners, participating in the market is not a simple matter of career survival or making profit. Whereas for some the processes of com-modification have allowed their knowledges and practices to flourish, for others the market provides a contingent ground upon which formerly un-thinkable personal and professional dreams can finally be realized. For Li, for example, the market is where traditional Chinese medicine can be po-sitioned as equal to biomedicine—not only in terms of market value, but more important, in demonstrating its clinical efficacy and in inventing health concepts and products for the cosmopolitan life. Unlike the socialist China where Li languished in his youth, or professional settings where he promoted Chinese medicine with limited success, the market is an arena where Li feels that he can express his thoughts (xiangfa) and articulate his dreams.

For Li Fengyi and others, repositioning Chinese medicine in a market economy is a matter of life and death for the profession, and in this man-ner they hold tenuously to the ideal of renxin renshu. Many other doc-tors and hospitals, however, have gained notoriety both in Shanghai and in other parts of China. Patients complain that hospitals and doctors have become too greedy and "heartless." Horror stories circulate through ru-mors and on the Internet of hospitals overcharging patients, refusing to treat patients who are unable to pay, or performing expensive and unnecessary medical procedures that compromise the patient's health. The doctor-patient relationship had reached rock bottom by 2005, at which time the Chinese Ministry of Health published a survey showing that 70 percent of healthcare professionals had received threats from disgruntled patients (Sina.com 2005).

Some of these threats turned fatal. On August 12, 2005, Dr. Dai Chunfu, a famous and well-respected practitioner of herbal medicine in Fujian Province, was hacked down with a machete by an angry patient while working at the Clinic of National Medicine (*guoyitang*) of the Fujian College of Traditional Chinese Medicine. The murderer was a twenty-nine-year-old man who had suffered various kinds of chronic illnesses, spending 200 thousand yuan along the way. Although he was not a patient of Dr. Dai's, he chose to assault him in public to vent his resentment toward doctors in general. The news of the attack spread through the Internet instantly. Astonishingly, an Internet survey revealed that 80 percent of the respondents were sympathetic to or even supportive of the murderer, 10 percent expressed neutral feelings, and only 10 percent condemned the murder (Xilu.com 2005). Many medical professionals expressed shock and dismay—shock at the violence and dismay that their reputation had plummeted so low since the SARS epidemic in 2003, during which they were briefly resurrected as heroes and saviors (Zhan 2005).

Even more ironic is the fact that the murder victim was a practitioner of traditional Chinese medicine who seemed to have exemplified renxin renshu. Dr. Dai was described as a cultured man skilled in playing traditional Chinese musical instruments, as well as in painting, calligraphy, and poetry (Xilu.com 2005). He often worked late into the evening, sometimes also skipping meals. When treating workers who had been laid off from their jobs, he would write down "laid off" (*xiagang*) to remind other doctors on the case not to pick unnecessarily expensive medication. Tragically, any medical expertise and ethics that Dr. Dai might have possessed did not save him from the general perception of doctors as the personification of greed.

Older practitioners on both sides of the Pacific have often argued that, for at least the last hundred years, the situation of traditional Chinese medicine, marginalized by biomedicine and entangled in shifting discourses of science and modernity, has been one of "life and death." Today in China "life and death" has taken on a much darker tone in the threats and actual beatings and killings of doctors by frustrated patients. But traditional Chinese medicine is not and does not need to be either soft in its knowledge production or heartless in its changing ethics. Processes of commodification have not simply fragmented or assimilated traditional Chinese medicine so that it looks more like biomedicine in its knowledge formation and ethics. Rationalization and fragmentation alone do not fully capture the complexity of the worlding of traditional Chinese medicine, and commodification is only one aspect—though an important one—of that story. More importantly, the role of commodification and entrepreneurship in the worlding of traditional Chinese medicine is not about creating a smooth circuit or an even field of circulation value across the Pacific or the globe. Instead, encounters with the biomedical mainstream have mediated and complicated the worlding of Chinese medicine by opening up new sites where professional knowledge, areas of expertise, and objectives of medical practice are all open to negotiation and contestation. Dreams and nightmares are made here.

Part Two

NEGOTIATIONS

Three

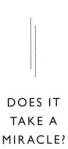

DOES IT
TAKE A
MIRACLE?

When Li Fengyi told me that he saw striking similarities between the American TV medical drama series *ER* and his own
everyday practice, I was at once surprised and fascinated. In
1998 and 1999 I worked with Li at the Jiren Clinic of Traditional Chinese Medicine, the private clinic that he cofounded
in 1994. Our discussion of *ER* and traditional Chinese medicine took place during a lunch break, when I was able to engage Li in conversations not directly related to cancers and
liver diseases—the two specialties for which he is famous in
Shanghai's traditional Chinese medical and biomedical cir-
cles. After I mentioned that I saw an episode, dubbed in Chinese on a local TV channel, Li told me that the same TV station was so inspired by the popularity of *ER* that they became
interested in developing a similar series—except that the
setting would not be the emergency room of a biomedical
hospital but rather a clinic of traditional Chinese medicine.
Pointing at the file cabinets behind him, Li continued with a
proud grin: "The folks at the TV station want me to provide
raw materials for the script! They prefer our clinic because it's
more eventful than the routines at a Western medicine clinic.
Take a look at these clinical journals—they are full of 'difficult
and unusual cases' [*yinan bingli*] we've solved. You don't have
to spice them up to create drama because each one of them is

a small 'clinical miracle' in itself! What could be a better way to advertise traditional Chinese medicine?"

Li is but one of the many "miracle workers" that I came to know in Shanghai and the San Francisco Bay Area. For those who have been socialized into traditional Chinese medicine—whether as practitioner, patient, or researcher—the ability to handle difficult clinical cases and, in particular, to achieve what mainstream biomedicine cannot is an unmistakable sign of professional accomplishment. At the memorial service of Zhao Zhenjing, a renowned practitioner and cancer specialist in San Francisco, Barbara Bernie spoke about Zhao in front of a diverse audience consisting of relatives, acupuncturists and herbalists, students of traditional Chinese medicine, former patients, biomedical professionals, and research scientists: "Dr. Zhao came to work at our teaching clinic [of traditional Chinese medicine] after he first arrived from China in 1985. He *always* asked for the most difficult cancer cases that Western doctors could not deal with. After he started his own clinic, he kept telling me, 'Send me the most challenging cases that you come across. I'll show people here what Chinese medicine can do!' He was able to help many patients who would have otherwise given up. He did so much to build the Chinese medicine community in San Francisco and to educate the general public! Dr. Zhao was very special." This narrative highlights the fact that, throughout his career in San Francisco, Zhao actively sought out and solved difficult cases that biomedicine had failed to treat. He was considered to be very special because of his own outstanding clinical knowledge and practice, and, more importantly, because he used his "miracle-making" abilities to craft a niche for traditional Chinese medicine within the biomedicine-centered healthcare system. In doing so he helped forge an inclusive, translocal community of traditional Chinese medicine that traveled across and was strengthened by networks that reached well beyond the local circle of practitioners. Zhao was in turn remembered in those terms.

From an ER-inspired TV drama in Shanghai to a memorial service in San Francisco, "miracles" take place in, and travel through, apparently disparate and yet connected settings. The fact that "clinical miracles" play central and vexed roles in constructing the translocal knowledges, identities, and communities of traditional Chinese medicine begs one immediate question: How has the everyday discourse and practice of traditional Chinese medicine become intimately connected with the production of the extraordinary?

In this chapter I examine the various kinds of encounters through which "miracles" are produced, as well as the ways in which differently situated people strategically invoke, interpret, and deploy these "miracles" to negotiate knowledge and authority in professional and broader social networks. In tracing the multiple trajectories and meanings of "clinical miracles" in the everyday discourse and practice of Chinese medicine, I show that it is precisely through the processes of marginalization and Othering in relation to "scientific," "biomedical" mainstreams that the clinical efficacy of traditional Chinese medicine becomes construed as "miracles." Furthermore, I argue that the marginality of traditional Chinese medicine is not a primordial structural position defined by a preexisting science proper. Instead of subscribing to a structuralist account of center and margin, I suggest that the marginality of Chinese medicine is constructed and constantly transformed through a set of uneven, interactive sociohistorical processes of knowledge formation, and at the same time marginality is itself a set of heterogeneous processes that mediate the transfiguration of various knowledges, identities, and communities that exceed the confines of the clinic.

In urban China and the United States herbal medicine and acupuncture are primarily used for conditions where biomedicine is less effective or ineffective. These conditions include, on the one hand, subhealth conditions such as allergies, pain syndromes, and other chronic illnesses (see chapter 1); on the other, life-threatening illnesses including certain types of cancers that cannot be removed through surgery and are resistant to radiation treatment and chemotherapy. Practitioners in Shanghai and San Francisco alike are quick to point out that many of their cases are "left over" by biomedicine. Often it is only after a patient has tried everything that "standard procedures" have to offer that they move on to traditional Chinese medicine, hoping for a miraculous cure.

Practitioners are, however, adamant that traditional Chinese medicine does more than passively fill in the blanks left by biomedicine. When demonstrating the medical legitimacy and authority of their own work and of traditional Chinese medicine at large, practitioners readily cite as a fact that, in everyday practice, traditional Chinese medicine is able to do what biomedicine cannot—sometimes even defying "death sentences" by biomedical doctors. Skeptics and opponents of traditional Chinese medicine, on the other hand, argue that these "clinical miracles" are too anecdotal or absurd to meet scientific norms. Yet, for their part, accomplished as well as aspiring practitioners of traditional Chinese medicine continue using "miraculous" clinical events to showcase clinical expertise and authority. They invoke "miracles" as affirmations of the clinical efficacy of traditional Chinese medicine, and even as testaments to its clinical superiority. In achieving what biomedicine cannot, "miracles" more than prove that traditional Chinese medicine works. These cases show that traditional Chinese medicine succeeds where biomedicine fails, thus making the comparison between the two medical practices part and parcel of the processes by which the clinical knowledge and authority of traditional Chinese medicine is constructed.

This comparison is by no means symmetrical. The fact that the everyday efficacy of traditional Chinese medicine is construed to be something out of the ordinary already assumes the normalized efficacy and the underlying scientistic "rationality" to which biomedicine readily lays claim. Yet even as the production of "clinical miracles" reinscribes the marginality and Otherness of traditional Chinese medicine, it opens up a contingent ground for negotiating fluid modes of constructing knowledges and authorities, and for participating in the production of science. At a time when Western medicine squarely grounds its authority in science even though its ties to biological sciences are historically recent and highly fraught (Starr 1982), "clinical miracles" as an ambiguous yet powerful source for medical knowledge and authority beg critical rethinking of what counts—and for whom it counts—as legitimate scientific practice. In other words, at stake in the production of "clinical miracles" is more than the legitimacy of an Other medicine, for our understandings and practices of science also turn out to be a contingent field for creative, interested play.

I do not assume a universalistic "science" or multiple, mutually exclusive "sciences" with predetermined parameters and boundaries. Nor do I restrict my analysis to communities of card-carrying scientists. Rather, by making obvious the processes by which knowledge, identity, and community are mutually constituted, I explore more participatory ways of envisioning and doing science. In what follows I show that what we have come to know as "traditional Chinese medicine" is a set of heterogeneous practices, discourses, and institutions produced through encounters and amid intricate relations with science and biomedicine; at the same time, the ongoing, translocal reconfiguration of the knowledges, identities, and communities of traditional Chinese medicine also transforms people's understandings and practices of science and biomedicine. I suggest that sociohistorically situated, shifting relations and boundaries between traditional Chinese medicine, science, and biomedicine play critical roles in producing, transforming, and reinscribing the marginality and Otherness of Chinese medicine.

Science and "Other" Knowledges

As has been repeatedly pointed out, "magic," "science," and "religion" form the three-cornered constellation that has shaped anthropological inquiries into the construction of knowledge, especially "Other" knowledges (e.g., Evans-Pritchard 1976 [1937]; Good 1994; Malinowski 1948 [1925]; Nader 1996; Tambiah 1990). In studying Other knowledges and in measuring them against science, anthropology has played a critical role in investigating and demarcating the boundaries of science, and the resulting boundary battles are "often arbitrary, rarely neutral, and always powerful" (Nader 1996:4). These boundary battles have also posed conceptual difficulties within anthropology. As Byron Good points out, the rationality debate in anthropology is often articulated in terms of "how we make sense of cultural views of the world that are not in accord with contemporary natural sciences" (1994:10).

This articulation itself may be the problem. Rationalist and relativist anthropologies have long battled along the lines of "rational" and "irrational," "knowledge" and "belief," "natural" and "cultural," "universal" and "local." In doing so, rationalists and relativists have reinscribed these lines even while contesting along them. In this section, I first give a brief review of how Bronislaw Malinowski and E. E. Evans-Pritchard, foundational figures in rationalist and relativist anthropological studies of knowledge and rationality, articulate their conceptions of science and its Others. I argue that these earlier anthropological inquiries into Other knowledges are themselves asymmetrical knowledge and identity productions that show the meanings and authorities of science to be relationally constructed. Second, I draw on Bruno Latour's critique of anthropological representations of Other knowledges to argue against using "rational" and "irrational," "knowledge" and "belief," "natural" and "cultural," "universal" and "local" to grid our inquiries into knowledge production. Instead, we need to critically analyze these categories as products of particular sociohistorical processes and to understand how differently situated players interpret, negotiate, and transform their meanings in interactive and creative ways.

Malinowski in *Magic, Science and Religion* (1948:26) addresses the problem of "primitive man's reason" by asking two questions. The first question,

"Can the 'primitive man' have any rational outlook?" is answered by Malinowski as follows: "Every primitive community is in possession of a considerable store of knowledge, based on experience and fashioned by reason." The second question is trickier. "Can this primitive knowledge be regarded as a rudimentary form of science or is it, on the contrary, radically different, a crude empiry, a body of practical and technical abilities, rules of thumb and rules of art having no theoretical value?" Under question here is not just "primitive knowledge" and the mind of "primitive man." Malinowski's formulation also offers, in passing as it were, a definition of "science"—not so much in terms of what it is as what it is *not*.

After momentarily dismissing the second question for being "epistemological rather than belonging to the study of man" (26), Malinowski returns to it with more vigor—this time laying out three possible definitions of "science" against which "primitive knowledge" might be measured. The first and "minimum" definition of "science" is "a body of rules and conceptions, based on experience and derived from it by logical inference, embodied in material achievements and in a fixed form of tradition and carried on by some sort of social organization" (34). The second definition states that "the rules of science must be laid down explicitly, open to control by experiment and critique by reason." After measuring "primitive knowledge" against the "minimum" definition of "science," Malinowski states that "there is no doubt that even the lowest savage communities have the beginnings of science." In invoking the second and narrower definition, he still concludes that "many of the principles of savage knowledge are scientific in this sense." But the temptation to draw the boundary between Us and Them, science and Other knowledges seems irresistible. Finally, Malinowski presents the third definition of "science": "If we applied another criterion yet, that of the really scientific attitude, the disinterested search for knowledge and for the understanding of causes and reasons, the answer [to the question whether primitive knowledge could be regarded as a rudimentary form of science] would certainly not be in a direct negative" (35). Although this final definition is the most stringent, even it, as Malinowski suggests, leaves open the possibility that "primitive knowledge" may be considered "scientific."

In articulating various conceptions and interpretations of science, Malinowski is as preoccupied with defining the "primitive mind" as with maintaining a sense of self-identity and producing a universalistic science. Moreover, not only is the identity of the European self at stake, but the unique professional identity of the anthropological scientist is also on the line: "There is . . . among the primitives, as every fieldworker well knows, the sociologist, the ideal informant, capable with marvelous accuracy and insight to give the *raison d'être,* the function and the organization of many a simpler institution in his tribe" (35).

In striving to fix the boundary between the "primitive man's reason" and "science," Malinowski's writing has highlighted, perhaps against his own intention, that what counts as science is open to interpretation and negotiation, and that the self-image of science/scientist is contingent upon the production of its Other. In the end Malinowski has to drop his quest, and he states that "the question . . . whether we should call it *science* or only *empirical and rational knowledge* is not of primary importance in this context" (35).

But this "question" continues to haunt anthropological investigations of Other knowledges. Evans-Pritchard in *Witchcraft, Oracles, and Magic among the Azande* (1976) approaches the muddled "it" from an angle that is more relativist rather than rationalist. For him the Zande practice of "witchcraft" makes sense—but only within its own cultural spatiality. His account of the Zande worldview is grounded in the constellation of "mystical notions," "common-sense notions," and "scientific notions." He asserts that the Azande understand the common sense of causation as clearly as do the Europeans: a Zande does not see a witch push over a granary but rather sees the termites gnawing away its supports (24). Yet the Azande also explain why a particular granary at a particular moment collapsed in terms of the mystical notion of "witchcraft" (22). In other words, the Azande use the notion of "witchcraft" to account for "coincidence," while the Europeans have no explanation of why chains of causation intersect at a certain time in a certain place (23). Therefore, as Richard Handler and Daniel Segal (1990) have argued, Evans-Pritchard's Azande have a common sense as sound as that of the Europeans, whereas their mystical notion of "witchcraft" is not an inferior but rather a supplementary explanation of concurrence.

In contrast to his relativistic approach to "mystical" and "common-sense" notions, "scientific notions" are for Evans-Pritchard, by definition, "European." He states that "we need not define scientific notions more clearly because Azande have none, or very few, according to where we draw the line between common sense and science" (229). Scientific knowledge is thus defined by the Azande's lack of it. In other words, although Evans-Pritchard uses "common sense" to unite human minds, he invokes "scientific notions" to mark the difference between Europeans and the Azande.

This cultural difference, moreover, is asymmetrical. He argues that "science developed out of common sense but was far more methodological and has better techniques of observation and reasoning" (229). Therefore the relation between "science" and "common sense," one having "developed out of" the other, is not only portrayed to be hierarchical but also implicitly evolutionary.

More important, "scientific notions" are where Evans-Pritchard grounds his own ethnographic authority (Handler and Segal 1990). An ethnographer is not just another European among the "primitives." Rather, his presence in the field is also that of a "scientist." While a layman may be uninformed and prejudiced, the anthropologist's preconceived ideas, by contrast, are "scientific" (Evans-Pritchard 1976:241). Evans-Pritchard asserts that he, the scientist, observes all the links of events, and that he judges correctly what he observes (229). Even though Evans-Pritchard claims to have let his fieldwork be guided by the Azande and their interest in "witchcraft," it is the presumed capacity for the science-minded ethnographer to explain all phenomena underlying Evans-Pritchard's interpretation of the Zande practice of "witchcraft."

The role of "scientific notions" in *Witchcraft* is thus twofold. First, the notions are presented as objective, authoritative criteria that relativize and affirm the specificity *and* rationality of the Zande worldview. Second, their presumed capacity to explain all phenomena forms an asymmetrical contrast with the Zande worldview, which makes sense only within its own cultural spatiality.

Many scholars have since contributed to the debate of science and Other knowledges and have taken it in various directions. I focus here on Latour's use of anthropological allegories in his explication of the two Great Divides (1993).[1] Having introduced anthropological concepts and ethnographic methods into social studies of scientists and their labs (Latour and Woolgar 1979), Latour takes an intellectual journey back to anthropology, and he draws on the insights from cultural and social studies of science to critically examine the conceptual framework of anthropology. He argues that in spite of its egalitarian goals anthropology, whether rationalist or relativist, has not achieved symmetry in the representations of non-European peoples and their knowledges. Rationalist accounts of knowledge and culture universalize particular strategies of reasoning, whereas relativist anthropology, in its various forms, is able to put cultures on apparently equal footing by reinscribing the omniscience and transcendence of the science in which anthropology grounds its own authority.

In trying to get beyond the two Great Divides Latour opposes the use of either the natural or the social as the ready-made, causal explanation of how science is constructed. He argues instead that nature and society-culture, as well as the division between these two realms, are constituted in the process of doing science; thus they are the results of, not the explanations for, how science is produced. Latour (1987) describes science as having the characteristics of strategically positioned "actor-networks," allying human and nonhuman actors and connecting them with interactive links through which controversies are settled and consensual knowledge is built into science. These networks extend well beyond the confines of the lab. They are forged by travelers who move across a wide range of social domains to accumulate human and nonhuman resources. It is noteworthy here that some of these translocal travelers cross the paths of "traditional cultures." Latour points out that this particular kind of path-crossing has played two critical roles in constructing science and rationality: making accusations about Other people's irrationality and appropriating Other knowledges.

First, in citing the anthropological staples of the Azande and of the Trobriand Islanders, Latour argues that it is by making accusations of the "primitive's" irrationality that European travelers construct and maintain their own sense of rationality. For these travelers, "rational" knowledge is presumed to be about natural phenomena and not about the people who describe them—that is, "Us" the Europeans. "Irrational" claims, in contrast, tell "very little about the phenomena and a lot about the people who persist in believing them" (1987:184). The divisions between knowledge and belief, rational and irrational, nature and culture are thus inextricably linked in the asymmetrical construction of knowledges and identities that distances Us from Them.

Second, Latour discusses the incident in which the French navigator La Pérouse appropriated the description of the local landscape by his Chinese fishermen informants in order to produce a map of Sakhalin Island and to include it in his map of the Pacific. In this case, "the *implicit* geography of the natives is made *explicit* by geographers; the *local* knowledge of the savages becomes the *universal* knowledge of the cartographers; the fuzzy, approximate and ungrounded *beliefs* of the locals are turned into a precise, certain, and justified *knowledge*" (1987:216). The European appropriation of Other knowledges is therefore integral to the production of universalistic science. As Latour notes: "Who includes and who is included, who localises and who is localised is not a cognitive or a cultural difference, but the result of a constant fight: Lapérouse was about to put Sakhalin on a map, but the South Pacific cannibals that stopped his travel put him on *their* map" (229).

By suggesting that the construction of Other knowledges is not outside of but rather part and parcel of the production of universalistic science and rationality, Latour's analysis of the accusation of irrationality and the appropriation of Other knowledges sheds light on the critical roles of "traditional cultures" in crafting and consolidating science. However, rather than critically engaging the "constant fight" for knowledges and identities as the ongoing process it is, Latour leans toward a Eurocentric position, and finds closure in qualifying the Azande, the Trobriand Islanders, and the Chinese as representatives of "the multitudes who *do not do science*" (1987:180; emphasis added). For him they are, after all, examples of "the people who are *not* part of the networks [of science], who fall through the mesh of the net" (180). In fact, by avoiding "the social" as the ready-made explanation of science and knowledge, Latour has altogether rejected the relevance of a wide range of "social actors" in producing science: "capitalism, the proletarian classes, the battle of the sexes, the struggle for the emancipation of races, Western culture, the strategies of wicked multinational corporations, the military establishment, the devious interests of professional lobbies, the race for prestige and rewards among scientists" (62). The roles of these social actors in shaping science, he states, are far-fetched and not pervasive enough, and these social actors are therefore not integral to the making of science. Thus, by excluding certain groups of people from the actor-networks of science, Latour inadvertently presumes a spatial image of science proper that has centers and margins drawn precisely along the lines of these "social actors." In his final analysis, with various Others safely placed outside of the networks of science, Latour's scientist emerges as a masculinist Eurocentric subject privileged to travel freely and forge strategic translocal networks. As Emily Martin points out, this scientist is "an accumulating, aggressive individual born of capitalism . . . resembling all too closely a Western businessman" (1994:135).

How would our conception of science change if, rather than assuming the scientist to be an implicitly masculinist and Eurocentric subject, we seriously reconsider and include the knowledge-making efforts by those who have conventionally been marginalized in or excluded from social analyses of science? Instead of depicting the trajectories of science as having origins located in the "West," what if we explore overlapping networks and processes with multiple points of departure, trajectories, and intersections? What if we follow the paths of those knowledge producers who are not (or not yet) card-carrying scientists, as they participate in, disrupt, realign, and even forge networks of science?

In this chapter I tell of a different way of traveling, a different assemblage of actor-networks, and the potentials for different kinds of subjectivity. Rather than assuming the "West" to be the normative referent for anthropological analyses of science, or viewing traditional Chinese medicine as a pure alternative to Western science and biomedicine, I examine the productions of knowledge, identity, and community in inextricable relations. In doing so I explore a more fluid and participatory conceptual framework for analyzing the production and practice of science. Whereas the South Pacific cannibals put an end to La Pérouse's journey, the practitioners of traditional Chinese medicine are still charting out new paths that reshape the topography of science.[2]

Producing Marginality

Marginalization is much more than the simple act of excluding traditional Chinese medicine from the proper domain of science and biomedicine. Marginality is not a stable structural position but rather the contingent outcome of a set of relational processes by which "traditional Chinese medicine," "biomedicine," and "science" are produced as their boundaries and relative positions are fought out. As part of the campaign in the 1950s to make traditional Chinese medicine more scientistic, the Shanghai Medical Bureau organized biomedical professionals to study and apprentice under senior practitioners of traditional Chinese medicine. This was not a one-way teacher-apprentice relationship, however. Not only did these biomedical professionals participate in the founding and administration of the Shanghai College of Traditional Chinese Medicine and its teaching hospitals, but also they went on to conduct laboratory research in an effort to demonstrate the scientific or material basis of medical concepts in Chinese medicine.

One of the most famous research projects was the research on "the material essence of kidney" (*shenbenzhi*), conducted by Dr. Shen Ziyin of Shanghai Medical University. In 1952 Shen graduated from the Shanghai

No. 1 Medical College, a biomedical institution later renamed Shanghai Medical University. As part of the campaign in 1955 described as "Western medicine learning from Chinese medicine" (*xiyi xue zhongyi*), Shen apprenticed under Jiang Chunhua, an accomplished herbalist. Shen went on to investigate what he calls the material basis of *shen,* an extremely complex concept in Chinese medicine that is commonly translated into "kidney" in biomedical terms. Experienced practitioners and educators of traditional Chinese medicine insist that shen is a concept with such complex functional, visceral, and metaphorical dimensions that it cannot be reduced to the anatomical kidney recognized by biomedicine. In everyday discourse and practice both inside and outside of Chinese medicine, however, shen is often conflated with the anatomical kidney, and this conflation is used by opponents of traditional Chinese medicine (as well as some of its young students) as evidence that Chinese medicine is vague or downright wrong about human anatomy (see chapter 2). Shen Ziyin, however, deals with the materiality of concepts in traditional Chinese medicine in a different way. Rather than dismissing shen as an imprecise version of "kidney," he claims to have found through laboratory research that the syndrome of kidney yang deficiency (*shenyangxuzheng*) is a malfunction of the hypothalamus (1976). In doing so, he disengages shen from the anatomical kidney and at the same time provides an alternative anatomicopathological explanation—in the form of the hypothalamus—for a classic syndrome in traditional Chinese medicine. Shen has built an illustrious career conducting biomedical research on traditional Chinese medicine, and he remains an ardent proponent of traditional Chinese medicine. However, his research is highly controversial among practitioners of traditional Chinese medicine in Shanghai. Some embrace the result and especially its perceived scientific authority, some envy the resources Shen's laboratory has at its disposal, and still others reject Shen's research for fragmenting and reducing Chinese medicine into something comprehensible to the biomedical ear.

The research on shenbenzhi is one example of how traditional Chinese medicine is marginalized—not by exclusion but through complex interactions and especially unequal negotiations with biomedical and bioscientific discourses, practices, and institutions. Whereas Shen's research affirms the validity of traditional Chinese medicine, it does so within the existing scope of science and biomedicine and by invoking the authority of laboratory research. On the one hand, the relation between biomedicine and science is assumed to be self-evident and goes uncontested: what could be more material or factual than the hypothalamus? On the other, the relation between traditional Chinese medicine and science is a lot more tenuous—a relation that is a subject of scrutiny by procedures, concepts, and standards acceptable to bioscience. Within these fields and relations of power, traditional Chinese medicine remains at best a provincial science.

Yet it is this provinciality that has allowed traditional Chinese medicine to be worlded as a "Chinese science." Beginning in the mid-1950s, proponents of the state campaign to promote traditional Chinese medicine and integrate it into the healthcare system argued that as a science—albeit a traditional, Chinese science—traditional Chinese medicine should be universalized and shared by the world. As some of the top Chinese natural scientists, including the geneticist Zhu Kezhen, contended, "Natural science is highly international. As soon as we form a scientific theory or make an invention, it becomes the treasure of humankind" (1954:3). Interestingly, the presumed universality of science and the exotic Otherness of traditional Chinese medicine, which are sources of ambiguity and even tension in traditional Chinese medicine, together allowed traditional Chinese medicine to be easily reoriented between the 1960s and the 1970s, the two decades that saw a major shift in the trajectories of the worlding of traditional Chinese medicine.

In the 1960s and early 1970s traditional Chinese medicine served, in the rhetoric of the time, *shijie renmin* or "people of the world." In practice, the worlding of traditional Chinese medicine was mainly oriented toward Africa, Latin America, and parts of Asia (see chapter 1). As the Soviet Union and the United States were also sending medical teams to the Third World, the encounters between "traditional Chinese medicine" and "biomedicine" were not about local-meets-universal but rather competing world-making projects. The worlding of traditional Chinese medicine not only drew on the universality and therefore legitimacy of science but, more important, it also succeeded in offering the proletariat of the world something that neither the Soviet medical teams nor those of the United States were able to offer—namely, acupuncture.

Beginning in the 1970s, mediated by shifts in geopolitical politics and a series of Sino-U.S. diplomatic events, acupuncture began to capture the fascination of the general public of the United States. Whereas in the 1960s many people in the United States saw acupuncture and herbal medicine as something exotic and "Oriental," today patient demand has prompted an increasing number of biomedical doctors to learn acupuncture and other alternative medicines. The mastery of alternative medicine is in fact becoming a constituent—if only a secondary one—of the biomedical professional's knowledge and authority. As a consequence the repertoire of biomedical practice is also undergoing profound changes.

Licensed acupuncturists are ambivalent, however, about the biomedical mainstream's enthusiasm over acupuncture and herbal medicine. As Barbara Bernie puts it: "Patients go to Western doctors for acupuncture because they think that these doctors are scientists and authorities of all kinds of medicine. What patients don't know is that the M.D. only needs to go through a few hundred hours of training to be allowed to practice acupuncture. A licensed acupuncturist has to have four years of training at an accredited college, pass the state licensing exam, and have their license renewed every year. *We* acupuncturists [i.e., licensed acupuncturists] are the real experts on what we do!" Like Barbara, while many acupuncturists enjoy their hard-won "mainstream" status they also worry about the field's appropriation, if not complete takeover, by the biomedical establishment.

Barbara and others are very much aware of the complexities and contradictions of interacting with biomedicine. For instance, the traditional Chinese medicine that the journalist James Reston physically experienced (as described in the introduction) was of a particular kind—and a recent invention at that. Called "acupuncture anesthesia," its invention in Shanghai during the 1960s brought acupuncture needles under the bright lights of the operating table. In the 1970s, acupuncture anesthesia was a standard procedure in most major hospitals in Shanghai, even though its inventors insisted that it was most suitable for rural healthcare in China and the Third World because it was efficient, low-cost, and easy to operate. Moreover, it was routinely performed in front of international visitors who were interested in medicine. By the late 1980s, however, acupuncture anesthesia had largely disappeared from both biomedical and traditional Chinese hospitals. The reason for this decline, I was told by acupuncturists and surgeons who once worked together to perform the procedure, was that it was "less effective" than biomedical techniques.[3] More importantly, according to these acupuncturists and surgeons, two decades of laboratory and clinical research had failed to produce any conclusive "scientific" explanation, as understood by biomedicine, of why and how acupuncture anesthesia works. At the end of the 1990s as postsocialist China worked to "get on track with the world"—or rather with the imaginaries of affluent Western Europe and North America—the state has placed a new emphasis on promoting sciences and technologies that would be considered "advanced" (*xianjin*) by "international standards." In the field of medicine, the development and importation of new biomedical techniques, equipment, and drugs has deepened the impression held by many medical professionals and patients that whereas biomedicine has progressed by leaps and bounds acupuncture anesthesia seems "stuck." By 1999 only one research project on acupuncture anesthesia remained active, and nowadays in Shanghai acupuncture anesthesia is no longer a clinical option. Thus, ironically, even though acupuncture anesthesia was itself the product of scientistic efforts, and even though it once spearheaded the worlding of traditional Chinese medicine, today it is becoming increasingly marginalized in relation to "international" bioscience and technologies.

The trajectory of acupuncture anesthesia is part of the broader socio-historical and institutional processes that have shaped the marginality of traditional Chinese medicine. During my fieldwork in Shanghai in 1998 and 1999 I frequently heard practitioners reminisce—as if speaking of lost wonders—about lost herbal formulas and acupuncture techniques as they gradually became crowded out by biomedical procedures. In a conversation with me, An Shidi and Weng Delian, two practitioners who trained in the 1950s, enumerated a wide range of traditional therapies that were going out of use, including treating internal illnesses with externally applied herbs; reducing infant fever with a special tuina technique; the utilization of highly toxic herbs, and so on. These therapies are considered too unreliable, illogical, or even dangerous by biomedical standards, and thus have been replaced by standard (e.g., biomedical) procedures. As Weng said to me:

> Our cohort has seen the ups and downs of Chinese medicine. It was hot in the late 1950s when we entered the Shanghai College of Traditional Chinese Medicine, but that wave died down by the time we graduated [in 1964]. When I was an intern, my mentor and I encountered a case of post-childbirth heatstroke. I asked my mentor why he didn't help. He told me that I was too naive—we weren't supposed to interfere unless invited by the Western doctors who were in charge. That patient died.

Then Chinese medicine was hot again in the 1970s. But, even during those periods when the government *was* paying attention to us, it was more symbolic than substantial. We never got quite as much financial or administrative support as Western medicine.

Now we don't even dare to deal with medical emergencies. When a patient dies in the emergency room of a Western medicine clinic, everybody is convinced that the patient is supposed to die. You'd be in big trouble if you used herbs and the patient did not get better. Patients and their relatives would make a big scene and name the biomedical drugs you are *supposed* to use. Just by word of mouth, people become well informed of what kind of cutting-edge antibiotics are available—even though they probably don't understand how they work or what exactly they are good for!

Others such as the San Francisco–based acupuncturist Jay Fitzgerald have confirmed Weng's observation about situations in the emergency room. Fitzgerald complained to me about the fact that in the emergency rooms of traditional Chinese hospitals in China one finds antibiotics rather than herbal teas. While on a tour in China in search of pure traditional Chinese medicine he caught a cold and developed a high fever. In spite of his illness he was excited at the prospect of visiting a traditional clinic in Shanghai. To his horror, however, instead of the herbal tea and acupuncture needles that he had expected he was given antibiotics through intravenous injection.

Thus the various configurations of the marginality of traditional Chinese medicine suggest that as scientism mediates the professionalization and transformation of Chinese medicine into a sensational, transnational phenomenon, it also redefines and even reduces the repertoire of traditional Chinese therapies. Moreover, authoritative discourses of science play important roles in delimiting the legitimate space of traditional Chinese medicine in relation to biomedicine, even as the changing contours, trajectories, and positions of traditional Chinese medicine call into question what counts as science, what counts as biomedicine, and what counts as traditional Chinese medicine. As I will show in the following section, it is only when the scope of scientific rationality and clinical efficacy is normalized in terms of the capabilities of biomedicine that the efficacy of traditional Chinese medicine is translated into something extraordinary and everyday practice becomes a site for the birth of "miracles."

From Clinical Success to "Miracles"

Clinical success has historically played an important role in the production of medical knowledge and practice. In China practitioners and scholars compiled collections of "medical cases" (*yi'an*) that documented personal experiences in everyday clinical practice, especially in efficacious diagnoses and treatments.[4] Until the first half of the twentieth century, the yi'an collections were important in Chinese medical writings and were commonly used as textbooks and references for practitioners.[5] Even today, aspiring practitioners use their teachers' clinical cases to enhance their own clinical skills.

Other than serving as raw material for yi'an, an efficacious clinical case sometimes played the much more dramatic role of career making. According to the memoir of He Shixi, a practitioner who was born in the first decade of the twentieth century, producing a sensational clinical case was how Zhu Nanshan launched his career as a renowned herbalist in Shanghai in the late nineteenth century and the early twentieth (He 1997). While still a young man, Zhu made a good living practicing medicine in his hometown in Jiangsu Province until he decided to move to Shanghai. Instead of attracting more business and living a better life, however, Zhu found himself without a clinic or much income. Depressed, he spent the better part of his days sitting at a teahouse. One day, the story goes, the handmaid of the mistress of the teahouse turned to Zhu for help because her son was suffering from an illness called *guzhang* ("drum distension") and none of the local healers was able to cure him. In order to help the son Zhu prescribed herbs for him. As He Shixi writes: "After taking Zhu's herbs for the first time, the patient sweated and defecated in a large amount. His body felt lighter, and his illness was halfway gone. The effect of the treatment was wonderful. Under Zhu's care, the patient completely recovered within a short period of time" (106). The mistress of the teahouse was so impressed by Zhu's efficacy that she spread the news to all of her customers. As a result Zhu became an instant success and eventually one of the top practitioners in Shanghai.

As remarkable as this story is, it does not imply that Zhu's success was entirely accidental. He Shixi points out that Zhu used a dosage five to six times the amount commonly prescribed (107). However, instead of seeing this as a deviation, He Shixi explains that Zhu's boldness was grounded in his ability to discern the clinical situation and his superb understanding of the ways of herbal medicine. In other words, although the incident itself was accidental, Zhu's success was not. Moreover, even though the initial success launched his career, Zhu came to represent the best of traditional Chinese medicine of the time only after his clinical efficacy was consistently proven.

Clinical success continues to be career defining in contemporary practices of traditional Chinese medicine in China and in the United States. In contrast to previous periods, however, clinical success in traditional Chinese medicine is often mediated by (and in turn marks) its marginality in relation to the biomedical mainstream. Indeed, the marginality of traditional Chinese medicine has transformed everyday efficacy into something out of the ordinary and at times even miraculous. For example, when I asked the herbalist Pang Panchi how she became a famous cancer specialist, she told me that it was "by coincidence." She tells the story as follows:

> My father was a traditional healer specializing in internal medicine. Our family practice was handed down from generation to generation. So I started with internal medicine. But in 1954 I started working at the No. 11 Hospital.[6] They did not have a gynecology department back then. So many female patients came to see me because I'm a woman. I remember that, in that first year, I had a patient who had ovarian cancer, and was undergoing radiation therapy. My colleagues in Western medicine said that her case was hopeless and even surgery would not help her. So she stopped medication and sat at home waiting to die. Her mother dragged her into my office. The mother got down on her knees and begged me to help her daughter. I started trying. The patient had severe lower-back pain, a large volume of watery vaginal discharge, and her tongue was pale. She had also given birth to three children. These were all signs of yin depletion. And I came to the conclusion that she had kidney deficiency [kidney as a yin organ], which caused damp heat and the stagnation of internal evils. I gave her a prescription. She did not get better. So I went to an older healer for help. He suggested a ready-made prescription in the Tang Dynasty medicine book *Qianjin Fang*. I changed a few herbs in the prescription and gave it to the patient. In a month, all her symptoms disappeared! She then went to the Women's Hospital in Shanghai to get a lab test. The report came out negative, and her tumor was gone! The news went around, and all sorts of cancer patients started to see me, hoping for miracles like this. Even the Cancer Hospital began

asking me to help with some of their cases. As I had more and more clinical experiences with cancer, I became a cancer specialist.

Pang is unequivocal and even proud of the fact that her career-defining clinical event was a "leftover" case from biomedicine, and the significance of this event lies in her success in defying a death sentence by her biomedical counterparts. The interaction and comparison with biomedicine is therefore integral to Pang's clinical success and translates it into "miracles." Yet this sense of the extraordinary also underscores the fact that instead of explaining or generalizing the mechanisms of Pang's treatment, the conceptual framework and technologies of biomedicine affirm Pang's efficacy only to the extent of confirming the result of her treatment in biomedical terms. The significance of Pang's "miracle" making thus remains ambiguous: she has accomplished what biomedicine cannot, and yet the rationality of her success is not accounted for—let alone normalized—by authoritative biomedical means. Also, unlike her predecessors such as Zhu Nanshan, Pang stresses that even after she became experienced in dealing with cancer her daily practice continued to have many cases that failed. As she said to me, "The Cancer Hospital only hands down to me cases they have given up on, and oftentimes it's simply too late for the patient." These failures, ironically, make the successes seem even more miraculous.

Like many practitioners in Shanghai, Pang is very much aware of the development of traditional Chinese medicine in the United States, and she is more hopeful about the future of Chinese medicine in California. Less obvious to her, perhaps, is that the stakes in producing "clinical miracles" are even higher in California. For many practitioners in California, clinical success is almost essential in making a living. Wendy Luo, an acupuncturist trained in Shanghai, recounted her experiences after immigrating to San Francisco in 1981 as follows:

> When I first started making a living here as an acupuncturist, many people did not know much about acupuncture and herbal medicine. Patients only came to me for illnesses that Western doctors could not cure. These were often very difficult cases. That's mostly true even today. And patients have very little patience—they would not want to come back if they did not see results quickly. That is a bit unfair—this is medicine, not magic! And why should people expect overnight cures from us, when they have had the illness for years and Western medicine could do nothing about them? But, anyway, I was lucky to soon realize that I had to

produce results, fast—I had to "wow" my patients so that they would spread my name.

I knew a senior colleague who came to the Bay Area around the same time. Back in China, he was very well known for effectively using toxic herbs to treat cancer. But he had problems here because the laws are more restrictive, and prescribing those herbs could get him into trouble. Also because of bad luck, he was not able to cure many patients. He lasted for a year and went back to China.

Many practitioners in the Bay Area have told me similarly complex stories of marginality and "miracle" making. Although at times the encounters with marginality seem disheartening and the pressure to produce "miracles" overwhelming, many practitioners also achieve clinical efficacy and use it to launch careers. Furthermore, as in the case of the deceased Dr. Zhao Zhenjing, "miracle-making" abilities and events facilitate efforts to engage biomedical communities and the general public and to promote Chinese medicine. Therefore, not only individual careers but also the development of translocal practices and communities of traditional Chinese medicine are at stake in the production of "clinical miracles." Back in Shanghai, Li Fengyi—like Zhao Zhenjing—also actively and decidedly engages the marginality of traditional Chinese medicine to perform "clinical miracles" and, in doing so, negotiates professional and broader knowledges, identities, and communities.

Making "Miracles," Transfiguring Science

The headquarters of the Jiren Clinic of Traditional Chinese Medicine is housed on the third floor of a gray concrete office building that belongs to a professional science and technology association. The building is located in the southwest corner of Shanghai—an area that since the 1950s has been the site of a number of major hospitals, including, among others, the Cancer Hospital, the Children's Hospital, Zhongshan Hospital of the Shanghai Medical University, and Longhua Hospital of the Shanghai University of Traditional Chinese Medicine (sutcm). In addition to the older buildings in the area, there is also something unmistakably new—namely, the clusters of unabashedly glistening "European-style" (*oushi*) apartment buildings that are much desired by Shanghai's emerging entrepreneurial and white-collar classes. These new apartments make the office building that hosts Jiren Clinic seem like an unwelcome reminder of the Mao era. There are, however, two activities that bring the building to life: the computer and informational technology lessons for local youths and the traditional Chinese medicine practice of Li Fengyi.

The door of Jiren Clinic opens into a small reception area and waiting room. A young female graduate from SUTCM is the receptionist, and she is often working on the computer where patient records are kept. The walls of the waiting room are covered with red silk banners embroidered with big yellow characters. Grateful patients have given these banners in praise of Li's medical ethics (yide) and his medical skills (yishu) (see chapter 2). A plastic Christmas tree decorated with red and gold ribbons stands in one corner. "My colleagues and students, and some of my former patients had a Christmas party here a few months ago," Li explained to me when he saw me marvel at the seemingly out-of-place and definitely out-of-season tree.

In the back of the waiting room is an office where two of Li's colleagues give medical consultations over the clinic's hotline. To the left is a meeting room where Li and his patients sit at a rectangular conference table. Unlike the crowded clinics at most local biomedical and traditional Chinese hospitals, where practitioners share offices and have desks squeezed back-to-back against each other, this room is enviably spacious and easily holds ten to fifteen people. Also unlike most local clinics, there are no laboratory materials or medical equipment in sight. There is, however, a wooden plate with the characters "love" (*ai*) and "kindness" (*shan*) inscribed in calligraphy by Master Hong Yi, the venerated Buddhist monk at the Temple of the Jade Buddha in Shanghai. Sometimes Li's Ph.D. advisees at SUTCM come in to use the desktop computer in the corner of the meeting room, where they write articles or look up information on the Internet.

Li tells me that originally he planned to have the patients sit in the waiting area for their turn to see him: when an individual's turn came up he would then interview that individual in his private office in the back of the meeting room. But the patients decided that they preferred gathering around the conference table so that they could chat in low voices and give out advice (sometimes wanted but more often not) to whomever was being diagnosed. During my visits to the clinic, Li and I would sit together at one end of the table with the patients gathered around us. In this venue it was interesting to note that Li stood out from his patients only by virtue of his white lab coat and the stack of prescription forms in front of him.

This smiling, unassuming man has had a life and career that, much like his practice, is marked by miracles. In 1966 at the beginning of the Cultural Revolution, Li's high school education was abruptly terminated when he and millions of other students were sent away from the city of Shanghai to work in rural China. In 1975 Li secured a rare opportunity to attend medical school at the Shanghai College of Traditional Chinese Medicine. Ironically, for Li the much-coveted opportunity to move back to Shanghai meant giving up his longtime interest in engineering. However, perhaps to his relief, Li was able to learn biomedicine at school. Founded in 1956 among China's first four state-run traditional Chinese medicine colleges, the Shanghai College is both admired and criticized for its commitment to teaching "two-fisted traditional Chinese medicine." This system includes *within* its scope biomedical concepts and techniques; in so doing it refers to, through contrast, other versions of "traditional Chinese medicine" as understood and taught by other colleges of traditional Chinese medicine in China that consider themselves more pure and orthodox.

On an average workday Li receives fifty to sixty patients. On my first visit to Jiren Clinic I arrived at 9:00 AM and already more than twenty patients were there. Some had seated themselves in the meeting room, while late arrivals waited their turn in the waiting area. The receptionist was occupied with entering data into the patients' records, which mainly held the history of diagnosis and the prescription, as well as summaries of the laboratory test results that patients obtained from larger medical institutions. In most cases the patients brought in their own records, but the computerized records ensured that the information would be available when patients were forgetful. Li is known in Shanghai for successfully treating cancers and liver diseases, and the majority of his patients suffered from these ailments. Most of the cancer patients at Li's clinic suffered from a few specific forms of the disease—notably late-stage cancers, cancers insensitive to chemotherapy and radiation treatment, and tumors that could not be surgically removed.

On that first day at the clinic I was struck by the fact that when diagnosing patients, Li used more than tongue and pulse diagnoses—trademark techniques of traditional Chinese medicine. He was also very comfortable with reading various lab reports and films, and with giving advice on surgery and biomedical medication. There were several patients who came in without any kind of medical record or physical exam, and Li gently chided them as he felt their pulses on the wrist. On another occasion, however, he refused to give a prescription to a woman who came in on behalf of her father, because, as Li explained to her, he could not examine the patient's tongue or feel his pulse.

The morning was almost over when a gaunt old man came in on the arm of a middle-aged man, whom I later found out was the older man's nephew and a former patient of Li's. The old man had lost ten kilograms within three months, had symptoms indicative of lung cancer (e.g., coughing, thick phlegm, and low fever in the afternoon), and had been refusing to get a biomedical exam. After checking the patient's tongue and pulse, Li said to me, "The patient has a thick, yellow coating on his tongue and the tip of the tongue is red. His pulse is wiry and rapid. In Chinese medicine, we call this condition 'ascending counter-flow of stomach qi' [*weiqi shangni*]. In Western medicine it is explained in terms of a large amount of sediments in the stomach. In most cases, this kind of condition turns out to be stomach or lung cancer." Then, turning toward the patient, Li said: "You have to get an endoscopy, and a CT scan or an MRI. Only then would I be able to give you a prescription that targets your specific problem. It would be irresponsible for me to give you herbs right now." Other patients also urged the old man, saying, "Western medicine too is science. It's available. So why don't you make use of it?"

Pointing at the nephew, Li said to me, "He found out a year ago that he had a malignant tumor on the back of his stomach which could not be surgically removed. Around the same time he was laid off from work. He did not want to live. His wife dragged him here. I convinced him to begin chemotherapy and take herbs and my formula medicines. His recent lab report came out negative!" Then, turning toward the nephew, Li said, "Don't worry about finding a new job. I'm working with my business associates to set up a network of traditional Chinese medicine clinics in downtown communities [*shequ*]. We will have three to five practitioners at each clinic to advertise preventive medicine and new health concepts that focus on prevention—Chinese medicine can also serve as a great preventive medicine! Maybe you can help us out at these clinics."

The day ended as Li saw off his last patient, a woman in her sixties equipped with a catheter unit. She had genital melanoma and underwent surgical removal two years ago. But the lesion would not heal after the operation. When Li paid her his first house call, her entire lower body was rotting away. One year of treatment with herbs and Li's own Chinese formula medicine (*zhongchengyao*) enabled her to walk again. She said to me with tears in her eyes, "Dr. Li is a miracle worker!"

It is noteworthy that Li's expertise in science and biomedicine is not outside of but rather integral to the medical repertoire that allows him to produce favorable clinical results and establish medical efficacy and authority. Li's patients, moreover, apparently are less concerned with the epistemological divisions that anthropologists see between biomedicine and traditional Chinese medicine than they are with what works for them (Farquhar 1999). And, after all, "Western medicine too is science."

Furthermore, unlike Pang who became a cancer specialist "by coincidence," Li seeks out liver diseases and cancers to be his specialties. Cancer and liver diseases are among the leading causes of death in Shanghai. However, biomedicine has not been effective in treating late-stage cancers, cancers resistant to chemotherapy and radiation, and tumors that cannot be surgically removed. Liver diseases, as Li and other practitioners have explained to me, can be even more difficult to treat because the intake of medication requires detoxification by the body, which is a function of the liver. Therefore, medication for liver diseases inevitably adds to the ailing liver's workload.

I once asked Li why he chose to specialize in cancers and liver diseases. In response he first said, half jokingly, "It's easy to become famous that way." Then he gave me a more serious answer: "Because these are 'big diseases' in biomedicine. How else can I make doctors of Western medicine take me seriously? They don't want to listen to you if you keep talking about tradition and culture. You have to play their game. And I want to get right at the center of the game." In seeking out medical cases for which biomedicine is ineffective or less effective, even if it means taking on what is left over by biomedicine, Li turns the marginality of traditional Chinese medicine into a vantage point from which he decidedly engages bioscientific medical practices and negotiates professional and broader knowledges, identities, and communities.

To be sure, Li's practice has many critics. Many biomedical doctors in Shanghai—especially oncologists and hepatologists—are ready to point out that he is, after all, a practitioner of "traditional," "Chinese" medicine. Meanwhile, some colleagues in traditional Chinese medicine criticize him for being too "Westernized" or "biomedical." Li is acutely aware of these criticisms. In response, he firmly grounds the legitimacy of his clinical practice in his ability to keep producing "clinical miracles." As he states, "I am not worried about others attacking me for what I do. My clinical results speak for themselves!"

But clinical results do not always speak for themselves. As Veronica Nelson, a young acupuncturist in San Francisco, puts it, "Herbs are sexy. But with our Western training we need scientific experiments to back them up." In both China and the United States, laboratory experiments and clinical trials on traditional Chinese medicine strive to follow the "standard procedures" by which biomedical experiments are performed. This particular way of conceiving of scientific experiments often poses conceptual and procedural difficulties for traditional Chinese medicine, such as in the case of acupuncture anesthesia. This does not mean, however, that traditional Chinese medicine always plays the passive subject that comes under the omniscient gaze of science. In fact, decades of experiments on traditional Chinese medicine have challenged the existing conceptual framework of science. Bob Miller, a physiologist who was part of the American Anesthesia Study Group in 1973, is now a professor emeritus at a large public university in the Southwest. Rather than scaling back on his research activities, he is currently designing experiments on the connection between qi and consciousness. This is an exciting project for him precisely because of the conceptual challenges it poses: "The conservative scientific hypothesis is that you can explain human behavior by brain function. That gives you a simple picture of the body as a machine. But that's not the whole picture. Qi, or life energy, just does not fit into this hypothesis. That's *shattering*. That's a big deal. That's bigger than a cure for cancer. That's the whole conceptual framework!"

Miller is one of the many who are enthusiastic about what they understand as a profound transformation that traditional Chinese medicine is bringing to more authoritative understandings and practices of science. Li Fengyi, for his part, takes part in producing and transforming science through classroom education. During a lecture for first-year students at SUTCM Li said, "We need to raise the level of the discussion of traditional Chinese medicine to the discussion of 'science.' Science is about rational explanations of nature, and these explanations are represented by scientific theory. No theory can be the exact reflection of reality because theories are always produced within and limited by specific historical periods. Yinyang and Five Element Theories, as we have discussed, are the conceptual basis of Chinese medicine and are examples of such theories. They are rational ways of understanding and coping with nature." In interpreting, reinscribing, and subverting modernist conceptions of science, nature, and rationality, Li not only rationalizes the conceptual basis of traditional Chinese medicine, but also transfigures science by placing traditional Chinese medicine firmly *within* the scope of scientific knowledge and practice. Not protoscience, not pseudoscience, not Chinese science—just science.

Many students find themselves captivated by Li's distinctive lecture style. During lectures he routinely uses his own clinical cases—or rather "clinical miracles"—to illustrate medical concepts and methods. Students are quick to tell me that they are willing to hear Li's views on science and medicine because these views come from a man with extraordinary clinical success. Some even seek out Li after class to discuss the question of science and the future of Chinese medicine. Li's ability to perform "clinical miracles" and to make them travel from clinic to classroom has contributed to his authority to speak creatively of and for science.

Evans-Pritchard reports that he had to let himself be guided by the Zande interest in "witchcraft" when he was in Zandeland, and when he was in Nuerland he became temporarily "cattle-minded" because that was the worldview of the Nuer (1976:242). For him being "cattle-minded" meant stepping outside of what he considered to be the realm of science and Us. The anthropologist's ability to be "cattle-minded" is thus grounded in the construction of the Great Divides—between science and nonscience, knowledge and belief, rational and irrational, universal and local, nature and culture, Us and Them.

Here I propose the potential advantage of being a little "miracle-minded" in our understandings and analyses of science. The multiple, creative, and sometimes contradictory ways in which differently situated people produce, invoke, and interpret the "clinical miracles" of traditional Chinese medicine remind us that the Great Divides are constructed through uneven and interactive sociohistorical processes, and are open to interested negotiations and transfigurations. Moreover, if "miracle workers" such as Li Fengyi can contest and transform these divides in everyday discourse and practice then we too can do so in our analyses of knowledge production.

I further suggest that to critically examine and move beyond the Great Divides we need to explore more fluid and participatory ways of envisioning, producing, and analyzing science, and we can begin by considering science as translocal, open-ended processes and networks for knowledge, identity, and community formation. In other words, we may think about the ways in which "science" is worlded and transformed. As I have described, in the everyday discourse and practice of traditional Chinese medicine—in particular through the production of "clinical miracles"—the recurring question of what counts as science proves to be inextricable from the question of who is authorized to define and craft science and rationality. The elusive answers to these questions are shaped by larger, transformative sociohistorical processes. At the same time, they also depend on the extent to which practitioners are able to successfully negotiate individual and collective knowledges and identities, as well as their abilities to forge and mobilize inclusive, translocal communities that extend beyond the immediate circle of local practitioners. The knowledges, identities, and communities of traditional Chinese medicine are constituted through shifting, overlapping processes and networks that render the boundaries between traditional Chinese medicine, science, and biomedicine anything but fixed or self-evident. In dismantling the Great Divides I hope we can further broaden the scope and means of anthropological inquiries into science by embracing the complexity in the ways of making knowledges and meanings.

Four

TRANSLATING
KNOWLEDGES

In this chapter I discuss cultural translation, both within a language and between languages, as a set of translocal processes and practices by which knowledges and identities are produced. I understand cultural translation as being irreducible to either the truthful representation of the meanings and logic of traditional Chinese medicine or its westernized forms. I suggest that translation is not a neutral process serving to "bridge" or "make sense of" differences between traditional Chinese medicine and biomedicine, East and West, tradition and science. Rather it is an uneven, formative practice that creates, privileges, and, in some cases, universalizes certain knowledges and meanings (Liu 1995; Pigg 2001; Rafael 1993). In what follows I show the ways in which differently situated people—practitioners, students, patients, and clinic visitors—construct knowledges and meanings through translational practices within the clinic and beyond.

Familiar Strangers

Shuguang Hospital is located on Pu'an Road, which is right off Huaihai Road. Huaihai is one of the busiest streets in downtown Shanghai, and it is famous for its upscale department stores, brand-name boutiques, restaurants, cafés, and sparkling office buildings. To reach Shuguang Hospital, I used to get off the bus or taxi at Huaihai Park at the intersection of Huaihai Road and Pu'an Road. There, in the early morning,

I often saw groups of seniors doing morning exercises. Their exercises included tai chi, sword dancing, and *yangge*, which was originally a celebratory dance of northern farmers but recently had gained popularity among the elderly in Shanghai as a healthy workout (Chen 2003). For the rest of the day the park was quite deserted, although on one corner there was a small café called the Glass House where I sometimes spent lunch breaks and wrote field notes.

The section of Pu'an Road between the park and the hospital is lined on one side with small, family-owned convenience stores selling snacks, soft drinks, flowers, and fruit baskets. These stores are strategically located for visitors of the hospital's inpatients. In Shanghai fruit baskets are popular gifts for occasions ranging from hospital visits to the Lunar New Year. There is also a small convenience store inside the walls of the hospital across the street. It is not much different from the other convenience stores, except that it also sells clay pots for cooking herbs.

There are two main buildings in the hospital compound. At the side of the street is the eleven-story clinic, which was completed in 1994. The entrance on the ground floor leads to the emergency area, and a ramp on each side of the building leads up to the clinic. The clinic is usually quite busy. During peak hours it was impossible for me to walk at my normal pace without bumping into someone. The visitors come from a wide range of age groups, the largest of which is the elderly—many of whom come in on their relatives' arms. Another eye-catching type is that of middle-aged and young women dressed in a loose-fitting, pastel-colored, translucent nightgown—a casual outfit popular among Shanghai's working and lower middle classes. These women, like the seniors, are mostly from the nearby residential neighborhood. Every once in a while a young woman in an elegant dress suit can be spotted in the crowd. She is likely to be a "Miss Office"—a nickname for the emerging class of women who hold clerical or managerial positions at nearby commercial corporations. For some doctors and nurses at the clinic, the fashionably dressed Miss Office is a somewhat unwelcome presence. They point out that, as the old residential clusters are demolished to make space for new office buildings, the Miss Office type has come to replace the elderly in the neighborhood. The problem, as one doctor loudly complained, is that "our regular elderly patients are moving away and these new, young ladies hardly ever get sick!"

Like any other comprehensive hospital in Shanghai, the first floor of the clinic has a reception desk in the center. Along the sides of the hall are the cashiers, along with two pharmacies—one traditional Chinese and one bio-medical. A big board behind the reception desk lists all of the departments in the building. Other than the various departments of traditional Chinese medicine, the clinic also hosts the Department of Cosmetic Surgery. As one of the newly established and most profitable departments in the hospital, cosmetic surgery offers liposuction, chemical removal of freckles, and eyelid modification to create a more European look.

The Department of Acupuncture (*zhenjiuke*) is located on the fourth floor of the clinic building. Also on this floor is the Department of General Internal Medicine (*puneike*). Like most traditional Chinese medicine clinics in Shanghai, the Department of General Internal Medicine, which specializes in herbal treatment of various internal disorders, is the biggest and strongest department at Shuguang. The Departments of Acupuncture and Internal Medicine are across the hallway from each other. The hallway between them forms a common waiting area, with four rows of pale green plastic chairs. During my internships at both departments I never saw all twenty-four seats occupied because most patients prefer standing around and hovering over the doctors in the treatment rooms. During peak hours the rooms get so packed that the nurses feel compelled to intervene and coax the crowd back into the hallway. Occasionally, people in Internal Medicine complain about the smell of *moxa* (mugwort leaf), which is sometimes burned as part of acupuncture treatment, drifting from across the hallway.[1] For the most part, however, the two departments coexist peacefully. The nurses from the two departments in particular have a habit of exchanging newspapers and gossip, although the doctors rarely socialize across departments.

There are five treatment rooms in the Department of Acupuncture. During my internship I worked in the treatment room headed by Dr. Huang Jixian, a chief doctor.[2] In Huang's treatment room a desk staffed by a nurse was placed next to the door. Entering patients were asked to hand their registration numbers and records to the nurse and then wait to be directed to one of the doctors. On the desk was a telephone (which seldom rang), as well as a huge pile of newspapers that the doctors and especially the nurses combed through everyday. The left side of the room was dominated by a large window, in front of which were placed several large pots of luscious orchids. Between the orchids were several ear, foot, hand, and full-body acupuncture models that occasionally were used to show students the precise locations of acupuncture points, especially the more obscure ones.

Under the window two desks were pressed back to back—one of which was used by Huang and the other by the resident doctor, Cynthia (who was introduced in chapter 1). Laid out neatly on the desks were diagnosis and prescription forms, official seals, stationery, and teacups. A chair was placed by the side of each desk, away from the window. Against the wall on the right-hand side of the entrance were a few chairs in mismatched styles ranging from large leather models to small wooden ones. On my first visit, I paused for a minute to figure out where to sit. I had been visiting clinics where the senior doctor sat in the tallest and most comfortable armchair, the intern sat in a slightly lower chair across the desk, and the patient was on a stool at the side of the desk. When Dr. Huang noticed my confusion she said, "At our place, you can sit wherever you want."

To the right of the door was a medical cabinet, on the top shelf of which were several electric therapeutic stimulators used in electroacupuncture. In this procedure the stimulator's wires are attached to the end of acupuncture needles, and the stimulator provides a low-voltage electric current that intensifies the stimulation of the acupuncture. During my stay at the clinic, I noticed a patient who preferred having the machine placed within his arm's reach during treatment so that he could adjust the electric current himself.

On the second shelf of the medical cabinet was a large tray of round glass cups used in the procedure of cupping. Cupping can be done either independently or in conjunction with acupuncture; when used with acupuncture, after the needles have been removed the acupuncturist places the glass cups on the acupuncture points that have just been needled. To put a cup in place, she lights a match inside the cup. As the air inside heats up and dissipates, she removes the match and quickly and firmly presses the cup against the patient's skin and leaves it there for five to fifteen minutes. It is quite a spectacle to see a patient with four or five glass cups attached to their bare skin, the removal of which often leaves red or purple marks that can last for days. In the past cupping was commonly used to treat cold syndromes. In recent years, however, it has enjoyed rising popularity in California and especially Hollywood. In 2004 the actress Gwyneth Paltrow was photographed with cupping marks on her back at a New York film premiere—an event that caused a brief media frenzy over cupping. Today in Shanghai and California alike cupping is a distinctively fashionable and relatively painless technique for not only pain relief but also weight loss.

On the cabinet's bottom shelf were stacked jars of moxa, cotton swabs, alcohol, and acupuncture needles. The most commonly used needles are the no. 30 needles, which are 40 millimeters in length and 0.3 millimeters in diameter. Longer needles are used for parts of the body where there are thick layers of fat or muscle. There are also a few other variations of acupuncture needles that are used for specific therapeutic techniques such as bleeding. Unlike the practice in the United States of using disposable needles, in the clinics in Shanghai the acupuncture needles are collected, disinfected, and reused.

Four wooden treatment tables, each covered with white linen sheets and pillows, were placed against the wall facing the treatment room entrance. Between the tables were two tall wooden armchairs. When there are not enough treatment tables to accommodate the patients, those who are having local acupuncture treatments, especially on the shoulders, arms, and legs, are asked to sit in these armchairs. The armchairs are also used when patients prefer to sit up.

In one corner of the room was a portable screen used to shield patients for privacy. I only saw it used once or twice. Although I never heard any complaints from patients, many international students were shocked at what they saw as the lack of privacy in these treatment rooms. I met Bryan Cai, an M.D. at the pain management center in one of San Francisco's major hospitals, when he went to Shanghai to study acupuncture. On the first day of his internship he expressed his astonishment: "I can't believe how little privacy there is here! There could be four or five patients in here at one time, and there is nothing separating them!" Students seemed to get used to this setting quickly, however, and they walked with Dr. Huang from one patient to the next as she worked with her needles and explained what she was doing.

When I arrived for my first visit I was struck by how crowded it was in the treatment room, even though there was only one patient being treated. It took me a few days to figure out that there were five regular doctors and nurses in the room—along with Dr. Huang, Cynthia, and two nurses there was also an intern, Xiao Yue, who was a fifth-year master's degree student at the Shanghai University of Traditional Chinese Medicine (SUTCM). Except for Xiao Yue, all of these staff members were women. As pointed out by Bridie Andrews (1996), historically in traditional Chinese medicine most herbalists were male. In contrast, because acupuncture and moxibustion were manual tasks considered inappropriate for the gentleman, women were allowed to develop clinical expertise in this area. Charlotte Furth (1999), furthermore, associates the historical gender asymmetry with the privileging of formal training in herbal medicine over informal training in acupuncture in Chinese medical discourses. Today the gender asymmetry between male herbalists and female acupuncturists is no longer so clear, although a number of acupuncturists in Shanghai have told me that their profession is seen as inferior to herbal medicine because they work with their hands. Dr. Huang, for example, told me that at the Shanghai College of Traditional Chinese medicine (SCTCM), from which she graduated in 1962, the major in acupuncture and tuina (therapeutic massage) was nicknamed *zhentuiban*. When pronounced in Shanghai dialect, zhentuiban is shorthand for "class of acupuncture and tuina" but also means "rather below par." In spite of these traditional divisions of labor, the gender composition of the staff in Huang's treatment room was quite unusual compared to the other acupuncture treatment rooms on the floor. In the Department of Acupuncture, as in most other acupuncture clinics in Shanghai today, the majority of senior doctors are male.

In addition to the regular staff, on my first visit to Huang's treatment room I met three international students and their English interpreter. I quickly learned that international students and visitors are a fixture on the scene, notably because SUTCM offers two short-term training programs in acupuncture. The beginner-level program runs from September to November, and the intermediate-level program runs from April to June. Both programs have internship components in which students are sent to the acupuncture departments at the university's teaching hospitals and several other affiliated hospitals. Some of these affiliated institutions are in fact biomedical hospitals that have strong acupuncture departments. In addition, some students contact the hospital directly in order to continue internships beyond their short-term programs at the university. To further complicate the composition of international students, those enrolled in the four-year International Education Program also come here for internships. Another group includes those who are making short visits for a few weeks or days at a time—most of whom are practitioners of acupuncture in the United States and Europe who come to the hospital to learn more about techniques. Finally, there are those who come for basic tours of the hospital. As noted in chapter 3, in the 1970s almost all of the healthcare professionals (along with a number of scientists) who visited Shanghai were taken on tours to witness the miracles of acupuncture, especially acupuncture anesthesia. At the end of the 1990s, however, traditional Chinese medicine was becoming a lucrative tourist attraction that appealed to a larger international tourist population than scientists and healthcare professionals. Tourist groups are encouraged to go to acupuncture and herbal medicine clinics where participants can receive diagnoses and treatments and purchase herbal products. Although most visitors at Shuguang remain scientists and healthcare professionals, the hospital is by no means immune to the overseas appeal and market potential of traditional Chinese medicine. In 2002 the hospital included in its clinic building a small museum of traditional Chinese medicine decorated with furniture in the style of the Qing Dynasty, and it began charging one hundred yuan (about twelve dollars) per person for a tour of the hospital.

Rather than being a foreign intrusion, international students and visitors are an integral component of the everyday practice at the Department of Acupuncture. Returning patients who are being treated for chronic illnesses sometimes joke good-naturedly about how they come for "traditional," "Chinese" therapies but instead are needled by foreigners.

Taking Notes

From the very start of my apprenticeship in the Department of Acupuncture, taking field notes was often a real challenge. It was quite unlike my experience at the Department of General Internal Medicine, where I apprenticed with Dr. Ma Zhongjie, a middle-aged herbalist who was in charge of training interns—often two at a time. Most of Ma's students, whether Chinese or international, came from the regular four-year program at SUTCM. Unlike the case with the short-term acupuncture students, fluency in Chinese is a prerequisite for the international students in the four-year program. As a result no interpreters were used in Ma's interactions with his students, most of whom were Koreans, Japanese, and overseas Chinese. During their shift with Dr. Ma the students sat around his desk and copied his diagnoses and prescriptions as he received patients one by one. When there was an interesting case, the students also came forward to check the patient's tongue and pulse. Ma always spoke out aloud as he wrote down on the clinical record the patient's chief complaints, previous medical history, and his diagnosis and prescription. Table 1 provides a sample clinical record for a first-time visitor (translated into English). As indicated by the categories on the clinical record, the diagnostic process incorporates concepts and techniques routinely used in biomedical practices. Moreover,

TABLE 1　Sample Clinical Record of a First-Time Patient

时间 (Date and time)	辩证分析 (Syndrome differentiation)
主诉 (Chief complaints)	治法 (Treatment principle and method)
病史 (Medical history)	方药 (或针灸穴位, 推拿方法) (Herbal prescription, or acupuncture points, or tuina methods)
望, 闻, 切 及体检 (Inspection, listening and smelling, pulse palpation, and physical exam)	诊断 (Diagnosis): 　(中) (Chinese medicine) 　　病名 (Disease/illness): 　　证型 (Syndrome) 　(西) (Western medicine) 　　病名 (Disease):
辅助检查 (Additional exams)	医嘱 (Physician's advice) 医生签名 (Physician's signature)

practitioners often authorize additional laboratory tests as they see fit. Shuguang Hospital is well equipped to perform a wide range of tests. At the time of my fieldwork, their proudest new acquisition was an imported MRI system.

After filling out the clinical record Ma passed it to one of the students, who then copied the prescription onto a form for the patient to present at the hospital's herbal pharmacy. Sometimes Ma also prescribed biomedical medications for the patient, and these were written down on a separate prescription form and taken to the biomedical pharmacy, which is also located in the hospital. For their own training purposes, the students copied Ma's diagnoses and prescriptions in their own notebooks. When there was a break, Ma would explain to the students the logic of his treatment, especially for difficult or unusual cases. Most of the time, however, the students took their notes home to compare with textbook cases.

The practice of copying the teacher's diagnosis and prescription is called *chaofang*, which literally means "copy the prescription." As noted by Judith

Farquhar (1994) and Volker Scheid (2002), prescription is at the very heart of the clinical practice of Chinese medicine. Senior practitioners have described in their memoirs that, until the institutionalization of traditional Chinese medicine, students had highly varied experiences with chaofang, for the teacher rarely explained for each case the logic of the treatment. Instead, students were expected to figure out their teacher's way of thinking. Those who could not, it is said, were considered unsuited for the profession because they could not think on their own and therefore could not be trusted to treat patients. Economic incentives formed another important way for teachers to withhold clinical knowledge from students (Hsu 1999; see also Herzfeld 2003; Yanagisako 2002). Although they rarely discuss it in their published memoirs, in everyday discourse senior practitioners acknowledge the saying that "the teacher who trains a disciple too well will starve to death."[3] Today in both China and the United States (albeit to different degrees) chaofang is still an indispensable pedagogical practice in both herbal medicine and acupuncture.[4] Many students and practitioners claim that "you don't know traditional Chinese medicine until you start chaofang."

The practice of chaofang at the Department of General Internal Medicine was so orderly that it turned out to be the ideal arrangement for me to take field notes. Dr. Ma was delighted by my detailed notes, although my fellow students were sometimes baffled by the fact that I wrote down things that obviously would do little in advancing my clinical knowledge and skills. My experience in the Department of Acupuncture was strikingly different, however, even though the pedagogical style also followed the chaofang model. Oftentimes there were several patients going through different stages of diagnosis and acupuncture treatment, lying side by side on the treatment tables without a screen separating them. Doctors and students walked from patient to patient, checking on the needles and discussing the cases. Sometimes it seemed like everybody was talking at the same time—doctors, students, patients, and the ever-present interpreter. All day long I would hear several different tongues—Mandarin Chinese, Shanghai dialect, and English—spoken all at once.

Amid the coming and going of patients and international students, Dr. Huang was the central person who held everything together in her treatment room. She was not only a seasoned practitioner but had also been engaged in international education and exchanges since the mid-1970s. The remainder of this chapter focuses on her and her daily interactions with students, patients, and visitors. In particular, I focus on the multiple ways in which she presents traditional Chinese medicine and translates medical and social knowledges within specific moments of clinical encounters.

Worlding "Tradition"

Dr. Huang is well liked by her colleagues and students. She has a disarming sense of humor and is calm even when everybody else around her is in a rush. In addition to my day-to-day interaction with her at the clinic, I had the opportunity to visit her at her house. Huang lives in one of the *shikumen* neighborhoods in the Jin'an District of Shanghai. Jin'an District was part of the old British and French Concessions, and the shikumen style was a typical architectural mode in Shanghai's foreign concessions in the 1920s and 1930s. Influenced by various types of European architecture, the shikumen style consists of rows of attached brick houses with trademark extensive stonework on the doorway and the facade. The original residents of these dwellings were mostly middle-class local Chinese who could not afford larger estates. During the Cultural Revolution, however, people who had been deprived of adequate housing, especially factory workers, started moving into these neighborhoods to share living space with the original residents. Nowadays it is still common to see several households occupy different floors and rooms of one shikumen house. Once a symbol of relative wealth and prestige, by the 1990s the shikumen style had lost much of its charm in the eyes of many Shanghainese. Some of the neighborhoods have been torn down to make space for subway and highway constructions, and the remainder are considered to be too crowded and unkempt.[5] Dr. Huang's family, for example, once owned the entire three-story house that she lives in. Now Dr. Huang and her husband occupy two rooms on one floor and share a kitchen with the four other families who moved in during the 1960s. At the time of my first visit, one of the other three families was leaving for a newly constructed "European-style" apartment purchased by the son, who had made a small fortune by starting a private shipping business.

It was at her dinner table that Huang first told me about how she became involved in acupuncture and in the international acupuncture programs. Coming from a middle-class family of intellectuals, she got into traditional Chinese medicine because of her interest in medicine combined with her feeling that, as a woman, she would be drawn to classical texts.[6] She graduated from the Shanghai College of Traditional Chinese Medicine in

1965, and she would have been assigned to a job in a rural area because of her family background, if the head of the acupuncture anesthesia program at Shuguang had not insisted that she was needed there. Still, Huang said that she did not get good training after graduation. As she said to me:

> Nowadays young doctors can go to seminars held once a week. When I graduated and entered the hospital, nobody cared. We lost a lot of time in the countryside. I was lucky because I only had to go to Shanghai's suburbs from time to time. Others were sent down to Anhui, Yunnan, and other poor rural provinces. We had nothing to do in the country-side. We called ourselves "*hongyaoshui* doctors" [hongyaoshui is a disinfecting solution commonly used in first aid]. There was no equip-ment, and we used to walk around the field looking for peasants who had been scratched or cut during work, which was pretty common, and apply hongyaoshui on the wounds. They thought we were strange be-cause these scratches and cuts were nothing to them. We, on the other hand, did not learn medical skills and were forgetting what we learned at school because of the lack of practice!

In 1976, after the founding of the International Training Center at the Shanghai College of Traditional Chinese Medicine, Huang started training international students who did internships at Shuguang Hospital. As she recalls:

> In 1976, when I started teaching international students, the guideline for the program [the International Acupuncture Training Center] was to train useful practitioners for Third World countries. When I first started, my students were all black. A lot of these students were the offspring of African government officials. They lived in fancy hotels and got paid for studying Chinese medicine. So it really took some devotion on our part to teach these students.
>
> I was almost not allowed to teach them because I came from a family of intellectuals and capitalists—not a working-class family. The govern-ment was very strict about class backgrounds back then. I remember that our hospital appointed a textile factory worker to sit by the door of the acupuncture clinic. She would check the backgrounds of the pa-tients. Those who did not come from "revolutionary backgrounds" [that is, factory workers, peasants, and soldiers] weren't allowed to interact with international students.

Huang's narrative is fraught with entangled racial and class imageries and allegories. Coming from an upper-middle-class family she feels alienated both by her dark-skinned African students and by the textile factory worker sitting at the door of her clinic. Her sense of alienation underscores the imaginary of a proletariat world that cuts across and reconfigures certain national, racial, and class boundaries while at the same time solidifying others.[7] Her particular position in this world, moreover, sharpens her sense of alienation rather than belonging.

Huang told me that when the Gang of Four was arrested in 1977, party cadres at the hospital were instructed to talk to foreign students to get "opinions from the world" on what had happened in China. At the same time, everybody else was told not to talk about it in front of foreigners. Beginning in the early 1980s, however, Huang noticed a drastic change in the composition of international students and, she claimed, their attitudes toward traditional Chinese medicine:

> In the 1980s, after Shanghai established close ties with the cities of Osaka and Yokohama, we began to see a lot of Japanese students. In recent years, however, my students are mostly white and come from North America and Europe. They pay out of their own pockets. We [sutcm and Shuguang Hospital] recruit mainly among nurses, physical therapists, anesthesiologists, medical doctors, and medical school students. We even take those who are biologists by trade. We also take practitioners of "traditional medicines"—every country has their own medical traditions. My international students ask more questions than my Chinese students! I'm so glad to see that they really care about traditional Chinese medicine.

While Huang stresses the shift in her students' racial, class, national, and medical backgrounds, she is equally insistent on her heightened awareness that these students have come to China to learn more about the "traditional" element in traditional Chinese medicine. Huang asserts that the students come to the acupuncture program looking for "differences." Other practitioners who are involved in international education share Huang's view. During meetings as well as informal conversations, they repeatedly point out that the international students did not come all the way to China to acquire knowledge and skills in Western medicine, for "their medical schools at home surely have the same if not better faculty and technological resources." This assertion is supported by reactions from international students. At the Department of Acupuncture at Shuguang Hospital, an acupuncturist who was well liked by patients earned a negative reputation among international students for using too many biomedical concepts in his pedagogical practice. Huang, in contrast, insists on explaining her clinical practice to international students using terms and concepts that she considers "traditional Chinese," even though her own everyday practice—including her conversations with patients—routinely incorporates biomedical concepts, techniques, and products. In the next section I describe some of the interactions between Dr. Huang, her students, and patients during a morning's work at the clinic.

Pains and Tremors

In the middle of November 1998 the weather in Shanghai turned cold and windy almost overnight. During this time the acupuncturists at Shuguang Hospital started to see an increase in the number of patients with facial paralysis. This was no less the case at Huang's clinic. On one morning during this period I arrived at the clinic to find it staffed by Dr. Huang, Cynthia, two nurses, and three international students. The students included Natalia, a nurse from Sweden; Adam, a recent college graduate from the United States; and Ellen, a pediatrician from South Africa. Although Ellen was a daughter of Chinese immigrants, she did not speak any Chinese. Ellen and Natalia were accompanied by Betty, an English interpreter who was a recent graduate of SUTCM.

Shortly after 9:00 the first patient arrived. Suffering from facial paralysis, he had come in for his third treatment in three days. During his first visit he told us that he was a recent graduate from Beijing University with a concentration in information technology, and he had just been hired by a foreign venture in the Pudong Development District in Shanghai. He had come down with a cold the previous week, and although he recovered from the cold quickly he found himself unable to use the muscles on the left side of his face. He was anxious to get well so that he could go back to work: the job market was highly competitive and he could not afford to fall behind. After checking his tongue and feeling his pulse, Dr. Huang decided to stick to the original treatment plan—"expel wind evil"—and she recorded it in the patient's clinical record. Natalia remarked that there had been quite a few cases of facial paralysis lately, to which Dr. Huang concurred by saying, "Yes, as soon as the wind starts blowing outside we see a lot of facial paralysis patients."

Huang then went on to explain the causes of facial paralysis. Betty translated her explanation, fumbling here and there for the right word. Both the patient and the students listened attentively as Dr. Huang stated, "In the old days, we would say that facial paralysis is caused by 'wind.' As you have already learned in your class (at the university), wind is one of the six excesses that cause illness. 'External wind' is the same as the commonsense concept of 'wind,' and we all know how our air is full of germs. In fact, a major type of facial paralysis—Bell's Palsy—is caused by viral infection. 'Internal wind' corresponds to today's notion of a stroke. Both can cause facial paralysis, but because one is external and the other is internal, the treatment would be different." The patient then asked, "I don't now about this wind or that wind. But my case really is viral, right?" Huang nodded. This brief exchange between them was not translated for the students.

With the students standing nearby, Dr. Huang began the patient's acupuncture treatment. She held ten needles between the ring finger and the middle finger of her left hand. With the first three fingers of her right hand she took each needle in turn, and using swift movements she inserted it into the acupuncture points on the patient's face, sometimes twisting the needle after the insertion in order to manipulate qi. When needling a few crucial points for the treatment, Dr. Huang asked the patient whether he "got it"; this refers to *deqi*—that is, to "get qi." For an acupuncture treatment to be effective, the needles need to be inserted at the right position, depth, and angle so that they come into direct contact with the flow of qi. In doing so acupuncture achieves its therapeutic purpose of manipulating and restoring qi to its normal level and properties.

Much of the deqi experience depends on the bodily contact between the patient and the acupuncturist. Over the course of my time in the clinic I heard students repeatedly ask Dr. Huang when they would know for sure the moment of deqi. Dr. Huang explained that the patient would experience numbness, heaviness, and soreness, so that the acupuncturist should pay attention to how the patient described their sensations. The acupuncturist, however, would also feel the qi of the patient through the needle. As Dr. Huang noted: "You would feel heavy and tight underneath your fingers. It's a two-way sensation, and you'll become familiar with it through practice." Indeed, Ellen yelped with joy after her first deqi experience.

After inserting the needles, all ten of them, Dr. Huang tilted her head to examine the layout of the needles to make sure that the arrangement looked neat. In response Natalia exclaimed, "Dr. Huang is an artist!" At that point, the second patient of the morning arrived. He was a man in his seventies, accompanied by two younger women who turned out to be his daughters. He walked in slowly, trembling along the way as if every step was a struggle. After instructing one of the nurses to attach some of the needles in the first patient to an electric current generator, Dr. Huang walked over to the old man. Together with the other nurse she helped him sit down. The old man had been seeing Dr. Huang until a year ago when she took a leave of absence to help set up an acupuncture clinic in Europe, and during that time he went without his acupuncture treatment. He told Huang that his tremors had gotten worse in the last few months after being hit by a bicycle. As Huang talked to the old man, Betty the interpreter came to her own conclusion. Without confirming with Dr. Huang, she turned around to the students and said, "He has Parkinson's."

The old man went on to tell Huang that he had also been suffering from constipation. Huang checked his tongue. She said to the students, "Look, his tongue is red and has a thick yellow coating. What does that indicate?" Natalia was the first to reply: "Internal damp heat?" Huang nodded approvingly. In the meantime, the patient had already positioned his left hand face up on the desk so that Huang could feel his pulse. Resting three fingers on his left wrist and then right, Huang stated: "His pulse is soggy and slippery—which again is an indication of dampness and qi stagnation." She then released the patient's wrist and urged the students to come forward and feel his pulse. As the students did so, she herself continued talking to the patient and his daughters, who were still complaining about the bike accident. After the students had felt the man's pulse and taken notes, Huang addressed them as follows:

> He was diagnosed with Parkinson's disease by our Department of Western International Medicine a few years ago. In Chinese medicine we diagnose this syndrome as "the stirring of liver wind, and phlegm stasis." There are three characteristics of Parkinson's disease: tremors, slowness in the movement, and stiffness in the movement. The explanation of Parkinson's disease by Western medicine corresponds to the explanation by Chinese medicine. In Western medicine it is explained in terms of a chemical imbalance, which is consistent with the concept of yin-yang balance in that they both stress dynamic rather than static balance. In Chinese medicine we think that older people tend to suffer from liver and kidney yin deficiency. Longstanding liver and kidney yin deficiency

can lead to excess in liver yang. The hyperactivity of liver yang can then stir up the liver wind, which is manifested in stiffness and trembling of the limbs. At the same time, we attribute the slowness in the movement to phlegm stasis.

As she spoke, she wrote on the patient's clinic record (see table 2).[8] Natalia then queried: "You said earlier that strokes are also caused by internal wind. Is that the same 'liver wind' that is associated with Parkinson's?" Huang was obviously delighted by the question, and said that indeed it was the same internal wind. Therefore, although the symptoms of facial paralysis caused by a stroke are very similar to those of facial paralysis caused by a viral infection, the treatment of stroke-related facial paralysis follows the treatment principle for Parkinson's. Rather than trying to expel the wind-evil, the treatment of Parkinson's disease and stroke-related facial paralysis both stress smoothing the liver and stopping the wind.

As the students, the interpreter, and Dr. Huang conversed, the patient walked over to one of the treatment tables and laid down on it. One of his daughters unbuttoned his shirt and cardigan and rolled up his trousers in preparation for acupuncture, which Ellen performed under the supervision of Dr. Huang. The patient and his daughters were obviously shocked when they tried to converse with Ellen and realized that she did not speak Chinese. They looked at each other and asked the nurses in a low voice where Ellen was from. Not wanting to appear dumbfounded by the sight of a woman who looked Chinese but did not speak the language, they quickly recovered. Nodding knowingly, one of the daughters concluded, "Ah, of course, she is a foreigner but of Chinese descent!"

After Huang had finished needling the points on the face, torso, arms, and hands of the patient, Ellen started needling the points on the patient's legs, beginning with yangling quan, the highest point, and moving down the leg. With the help of Dr. Huang, the interpreter, and body language, she and the patient communicated about how he felt about her needling—too deep or too shallow, too much stimulation or not enough. In the meantime, Natalia started telling Dr. Huang that an acupuncturist at a different hospital used different points for the treatment of Parkinson's disease. Both Dr. Huang and Cynthia were fascinated by Natalia's remarks, and they asked her in detail about the exact points the other acupuncturist had used. Before they could finish the conversation, however, two new patients walked in and Dr. Huang went over to greet them.

TABLE 2   Sample Clinical Record of a Returning Patient

复诊病史 (Returning patient's history) *See previous record. Tremors have worsened since September.*	治则治法 (Treatment principle and method) *Smooth the liver and calm the wind. Channel out phlegm dampness.*
舌象(Tongue) *Red tongue, yellow coating*	方名(Acupuncture points) *Baihui* (GV 20), *tianchi* (CV 24), *quchi* (LI 11), *waiguan* (TB 5), *hegu* (LI 4), *yanglingquan* (GB 34), *zusanli* (ST 36), *sanyinjiao* (SP 6), *taixi* (KI 3), *taichong* (LV 3)
脉象 (Pulse) *Soggy, slippery*	
实验室检查 (Laboratory tests)	方药 (Patent medicine)
辩证分析 (Syndrome differentiation) *The patient is over sixty. Liver and kidney yin deficiency. Yang excess caused by yin deficiency. Liver wind is stirred. Phlegm stasis.*	诊断 (病名) (Diagnosis: Name of illness/disease) *Parkinson's*

By the time the morning was nearly over, twelve patients had been treated—five of whom suffered from facial paralysis. At one point Huang said jokingly to the students, "Now you are all experts in facial paralysis!" In response Natalia stated, "But we hardly ever get any facial paralysis cases in our countries!" She then went on to ask Dr. Huang what points could be used in the treatment of skin allergies and diabetes, which she said were more commonly seen conditions at her clinic. Huang described the commonly used points for skin allergies, but then recommended herbal treatment for diabetes: "In the old days, people used to apply acupuncture to disorders in the internal organs as well as skeletal-muscular problems. These days, acupuncture is more and more restricted to the treatment of skeletal-muscular disorders, especially pain syndromes."

During this conversation the patients, upon hearing Natalia saying that facial paralysis (caused by viral infection) was uncommon in her country, began their own discussion about why they were all suffering from it. Someone said, "Chinese viruses are especially potent!" Another said, "Facial paralysis is the byproduct of Chinese culture." The first patient then continued, "The Chinese have weaker bodies. The foreigners eat better, get better nutrition, and have better immune systems." Others concurred, "Yes, the foreigners have stronger immune systems."

One patient, whose needles had been removed, walked over to another to admire the needles in his face. He was a journalist in his early forties—like Li Fengyi he belonged to the generation that came of age during the Cultural Revolution. He said to the other patients, "We are comrades in suffering!" Then, continuing the conversation about the immune system, he said, "The high rate of facial paralysis in China is a political problem. We lived through so many government campaigns: land reform, the Cultural Revolution . . . People are always nervous and stressed out. That's why our immune systems are weakened." Another patient agreed, "Yeah, one campaign after another—we all suffered."

Someone turned to Dr. Huang and said, "Dr. Huang, you know this too. From now on you should ask your facial paralysis patients whether they are under constant pressure." Dr. Huang answered good-naturedly, "I used to pay attention to patients' professional occupation. But I'll pay attention to their stress level as well." An older patient noticed that Betty had been whispering to the students, who were so intrigued by the conversation that they asked Betty to translate it. At this the older patient added sheepishly, "We were no longer stressed after Deng Xiaoping took over." The journalist, however, took the opportunity to ask the students if they knew about the Cultural Revolution. Adam said that he knew an acupuncturist who was sent to a remote rural area and was stranded there for seventeen years. "It was horrible," Adam said. He added that the acupuncturist eventually went to the United States and was practicing acupuncture there.

As lunchtime approached, the patients left one after another. The journalist hung around long after his own treatment was finished, and he was the last to leave. Dr. Huang and Betty started discussing the depth of insertions. Huang said, "When I was in Europe I used 1-*cun* needles, and the insertions I made were a lot shallower than what I would normally do for patients here. It seems that foreigners have much lower tolerance for pain—some women cry during acupuncture! When I first came back, I used shallow insertions as well. But my patients told me that they could

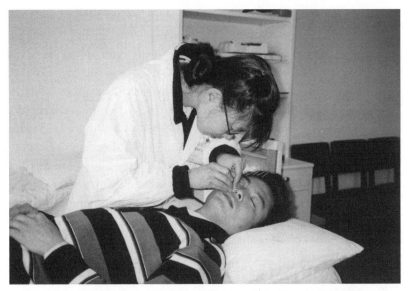

An international student treats a patient with facial paralysis, Shuguang Hospital, Shanghai. Photo by the author.

not feel anything." Upon hearing Huang's story, the journalist said, "See what I mean? We Chinese are really good at enduring pain."

In Huang's conversations with her students and patients she took disease categories and reasoning strategies commonly used in biomedicine and skillfully wove them together with therapeutic concepts and practices unique to traditional Chinese medicine. She accomplished this first of all by readily invoking biomedical understandings of disease and treatment familiar to doctors, students, and, perhaps to a lesser extent, patients. Diagnostic categories such as "Parkinson's disease" were integral to Huang's everyday clinical practice: not as universals but as referents for translating concepts and practices that she and her students deemed "traditional Chinese." While invoking biomedical concepts, Huang also avoided letting them singularly define "what is really going on." She did not subscribe to the language of biomedicine as the only authoritative means of constructing and representing clinical reality. Instead, she privileged biomedical concepts as heuristic and translational referents in communicating with both patients and students. In doing so, she "relativized" biomedicine without completely rejecting or embracing it. Second, Huang referred to but did not dwell on biomedical concepts and practices in her pedagogy. Instead she emphasized the unique qualities of the therapeutic concepts and practices of traditional Chinese medicine, as defined in terms of their *differences* from and even incomparability with biomedicine. In other words, it was by drawing on discourses of difference and through everyday translational practices that Huang and her students co-constructed a distinctively "traditional," "Chinese" medicine. Finally, the everyday translocal encounters and translational practices not only project what was "traditional Chinese medicine" to international students but also provided occasions for doctors, patients, and students to articulate the cultural politics of being Chinese. For example, sensations of pain quickly turned into reflections on the social body, and discussions of the immune system became poignant social commentaries on the sociopolitical conditions in China. Indeed, the embodied experience of being Chinese was sharpened by the bodily presence of foreign students.

Talking "Science"

In December the international students at the International Acupuncture Education Program completed their training and departed. Short-term visitors, however, still showed up at the Department of Acupuncture quite frequently. Many of these visitors were healthcare professionals who were curious about traditional Chinese medicine or had some training in it. One of these visitors was Dr. Bai, M.D., a Chinese American who came from an industrial city in the American Midwest.

As a U.S.-trained M.D. Dr. Bai practiced internal medicine and geriatrics at his own clinic. He spoke both English and Mandarin Chinese fluently. He told me that this was his first trip to China, and the main purpose for the trip was to look for treatments of diseases where Western medicine is ineffective. Pointing at one of the patients in the room, he said, "Parkinson's, for example. We use a lot of steroids, but the side effects are really bad." He had been studying with an acupuncturist in his city for two years, but he did not practice herbal medicine because it was difficult for him to obtain herbs. He did not practice moxibustion because it set off the fire alarms in his clinic, and cupping was a problem because his patients would complain about the bruising.

Upon hearing our conversation, Dr. Huang suggested that Dr. Bai explain to his patients how cupping works. He smiled politely, but did not say anything. But his smile was replaced by a look of shock when one of the patients on the treatment tables started snoring. Fighting back a smile, Huang asked Bai what diseases he would treat with acupuncture in his clinic. In response Bai listed bursitis, tendonitis, sprains, lower back pain, and so on. Bai then asked Huang whether numbness in the fingers could be treated with acupuncture, and Huang replied that it would depend on the cause. For example, if the cause was neuritis in the nerve ending then the numbness could be treated by acupuncture. Bai was obviously impressed with Huang's knowledge of technical terms in biomedicine, and he warmed up to the conversation.

Bai then asked about Parkinson's disease, noting that "Western medicine really does not have good treatment for Parkinson's. Some teaching hospitals of big medical schools have the technology and equipment for three-dimensional CT and neurosurgery, but these are still experimental." In response, Huang stated: "There are surgical procedures available at Huashan Hospital in Shanghai as well.[9] It's also still experimental. For the Chinese, going through surgery is a big deal because it hurts *yuanqi* (the body's 'primordial qi'). That's why the Chinese are especially cautious about surgery and avoid it as long as they can." Bai answered, "Yes. And brain surgery is even more complicated. For Parkinson's disease, the surgery has to get into the center of the brain." Huang nodded, "So, yes, people are even more cautious about brain surgery. Acupuncture, on the other hand, helps reduce muscular tension and therefore relieve the patient's state of intensity. So the patient would not have to take as much steroid medication."

At that point, the wife of the Parkinson's patient joined the conversation, "My old man actually went to Huashan Hospital, and he saw one case where the person who underwent surgery recovered from Parkinson's. But he is afraid of surgery, and prefers acupuncture. His condition has really improved a lot! Besides, the surgery would cost seventy to eighty thousand yuan (nearly ten thousand dollars in 1998). Now that the work unit no longer pays for it, we cannot afford an expensive surgery like this!"

Bai wanted to know more about scientific research on acupuncture, and Huang replied that there hadn't been any real breakthrough. Turning to me, she said, "Like I told you yesterday, the researchers are not able to explain the physical basis of the meridians." Bai then asked if the meridian system is related to the Western notion of the nervous system. Huang said, "No, we traditional Chinese doctors don't talk about the nervous system. The meridians are completely different from the nervous system: experiments have already shown that the body's response to acupuncture has a speed different from the speed of neural transmission."

Bai pressed on, however, by asking whether deqi was related to the nervous system. Huang's answer was again in the negative. She continued as Bai listened attentively: "Again, this is something that cannot be measured by machines. Westerners want everything to be accurate, and the biggest difficulty they have with Chinese medicine is that it cannot be quantified. I have taught many international students, so I know this. Whenever you tell them a certain treatment is effective, they would ask what the efficacy rate is. If you teach them how to twirl the needle, they would ask how many times they should twirl. In fact, none of this is fixed or easily quantified."

As she did in her interactions with international students, Huang readily invoked biomedical terminology in her conversation with Bai. Moreover, her display of biomedical and bioscientific knowledge here served an additional purpose. In the beginning Dr. Bai hardly talked to Dr. Huang. In fact, most of the exchange took place between him and me—the anthropologist from Stanford. He quickly became interested in talking to Huang, however, as soon as she proved to him that, like him, she could "talk science." Huang used her fluency in biomedical vocabulary to gain leverage and authority in her interaction with Bai, the U.S.-trained medical doctor. Moreover, by demonstrating that she was well read in scientific literature and that her knowledge of scientific experiments was up to date, she managed to argue that the conception of the body in traditional Chinese medicine is not inferior to but simply different from biomedicine. For her, the meridian system is not simply a protoscientific variation of the biomedical conception of the nervous system but rather something radically different. In other words, Huang's strategic display of her scientific knowledge helped strengthen her argument about the irreducible differences. Finally, Huang also used her expertise in bioscientific knowledge for a gentle critique of the reductionist and universalizing tendency in biomedicine. Citing results from laboratory experiments on the meridian system, she argued that the passion of westerners for numbers undermined their attempt to understand traditional Chinese medicine. In her opinion, biomedicine failed to account for the workings of traditional Chinese medicine precisely because of its undue faith in its universalizing power.

In communicating with international students and visitors, Huang does not explain traditional Chinese medicine in biomedical terms. Although biomedical concepts and techniques are constitutive of her everyday acupuncture practice, Huang is extremely skillful and purposeful in using her repertoire of clinical knowledge and expertise to question the presumed universality of biomedical discourses—and thereby the monopolistic claim to science by biomedicine. At the same time, Huang does not seek to deliver the "logic" of traditional Chinese medicine as prepackaged, self-explanatory goods. Instead she carefully negotiates terms of difference by knowing exactly when to forge connection and when to insist on being incommensurable. She crafts a distinctively traditional, Chinese medicine through strategic and mobile positioning vis-à-vis biomedicine in everyday translational practices to form a kind of traditional Chinese medicine that is at once different from and familiar to biomedicine. In doing so she constantly nudges her interlocutors—whether students or visitors, Chinese or foreign—to rethink the taken-for-granted boundary of and hierarchy between biomedicine and Chinese medicine.

Huang is but one of the many practitioners of traditional Chinese medicine who day in and day out take part in the translational practices between doctors and patients, teachers and students, practitioners of traditional Chinese medicine and biomedicine. Many practitioners are savvy travelers across disparate institutional sites, especially in hospitals, clinics, and classrooms, and at conferences on both traditional Chinese medicine and biomedicine. They also cross national boundaries to attend international conferences and workshops, negotiate and arrange joint programs, and visit families, teachers, or students (see chapter 6). Whereas these are obvious cases, dense moments of translocal encounters occur every day at institutional sites as small as the Department of Acupuncture at Shuguang Hospital. And it is also within these effervescent moments that Chinese medicine is translated, reinterpreted, challenged, and performed—that is, worlded. Not all practitioners are as skillful as Huang in navigating the shifting translocal fields of knowledge and power. Yet all engage in some kind of translation that constantly probes the taken-for-granted boundaries and order of authorities. Translation is all too mundane and yet at the same time it cannot be more critical for the knowledge production of Chinese medicine.

Translocal encounters and translational practices are not external to the "core" of traditional Chinese medicine; rather, these are everyday processes and practices by which the very knowledges and meanings of traditional Chinese medicine are relationally produced, negotiated, contested, and legitimized. As argued by Lydia Liu (1995:26), cultural translation is the very site of encounter where irreducible differences are fought out, authorities invoked and challenged, and ambiguities dissolved or created. A critical study of the cultural translation of traditional Chinese medicine is neither a rationalist nor a relativist project, but it might ask the question of how tradition, science, and the politics of difference are worlded through translations.

Part Three

DISLOCATIONS

Five

$$\|$$

ENGENDERING
FAMILIES AND
KNOWLEDGES,
SIDEWAYS

In 1938 the Western-trained physician Wong Chimin founded the Museum of the History of Chinese Medicine (Zhongguo Yishi Bowuguan). Having coauthored, with Wu Lien-The, the first book on the history of medicine in China, Wong decided to develop the museum as part of his effort to showcase China's robust history of medical practice, which had been so routinely ignored by European medical historians.[1] In 1959 the museum was relocated to the campus of the recently founded Shanghai College of Traditional Chinese Medicine (SCTCM), and the collection housed there grew over the years. Today, a visit to the Museum is required of all students at the Shanghai University of Traditional Chinese Medicine (SUTCM)—Chinese and international, full-time students and short-term trainees.

On December 31, 1998, I was given a tour of the museum by Chen Maoren, a senior practitioner who taught at the university. An assistant at the museum accompanied us. The tour began with the etching of a Han Dynasty stele depicting Shennong, the "Divine Farmer," who is the mythical ancestor of agriculture and herbal medicine.[2] From there we examined a display of material history, including therapeutic instruments, illustrations of techniques, medical textbooks, acupuncture models, and biographies of famous healers.

Arranged in chronological order, the exhibition emphasized antiquity, continuity, and progress: forty-four surgical tools from the Qing Dynasty, for example, were meticulously arranged and displayed as a demonstration of the existence of a Chinese tradition in "surgery" (*waike*) and as a silent rebuke of any argument to the contrary.[3]

Among the museum's exhibits I was most captivated by the glass display cases that housed written prescriptions, medicine boxes, and calligraphy and paintings by some of the famous literati doctors (*ruyi*) who worked in the neighboring provinces of Jiangsu and Zhejiang in the second half of the nineteenth century. With the emergence of Shanghai as a colonial treaty port and cosmopolitan city around that time, many of these practitioners had moved their families and practices to the burgeoning city.[4] As we gazed at the elegant calligraphy and paintings, Chen told me that the sons, grandsons, and students of these practitioners helped found SCTCM and, in some cases, still held administrative and teaching positions there. Today, the administration at the university, as well as many local practitioners, consider these literati doctors among the founding fathers of the community of traditional Chinese medicine in Shanghai.

Chen himself came from a famous family of herbalists who had passed on their knowledge and practice for four generations through their male line. When he graduated from high school in 1958, he had intended to go into biomedicine, which he considered "better" than Chinese medicine. However, local educational and healthcare officials urged him to study as a disciple under his father and become an herbalist instead. Ironically, even though official state discourses branded family practice and discipleship as part of the backward elements of Chinese medicine that needed to be modernized through standardization, the roles played by family succession and discipleship were important in the institutionalization of Chinese medicine. Indeed, it was through state-sponsored small study groups and discipleships that biomedical professionals were retrained so that they could help establish and manage the large-scale colleges and hospitals of traditional Chinese medicine. In addition, healthcare officials at various levels recruited the offspring of families of traditional Chinese medicine to continue their families' practices. After many conversations with these officials, Chen reluctantly agreed to go to SCTCM and study under his father, who had by then become a member of the faculty.

Chen's experience is shared by a number of other male practitioners of his generation: whereas some carried on their families' trade willingly, others had to be persuaded by officials, administrators, and family members. These reluctant heirs, however, have emerged as successful practitioners and teachers in their own right. Today certain surnames—such as Ding, He, Gu, and so on—are still highly respected by practitioners and sought after by experienced patients. Acknowledging the cultural capital of a prestigious surname, practitioners who have inherited medical knowledges and practices from their families (and, occasionally, those who have not) advertise themselves as such regardless of the various career dreams and goals to which they might once have aspired.

Among the current students at SUTCM, a classmate who comes from a family of traditional Chinese medicine practitioners continues to arouse much interest and even envy. Many students remain convinced that such teachers would reserve the best of their medical knowledge for their own children and a few chosen disciples. However, the few students who come from families of Chinese medicine often placate their classmates by insisting that their family legacy is "nothing more than a few old books." Rather than having their family legacy and career path combined into one and laid out before them, many young heirs face the same dilemma as those of Chen's generation. Chen's own son is one of them. At the end of the tour, Chen told me and the museum assistant that his son was planning to quit his current job and go back to school with the aim of attending one of Shanghai's two biomedical universities to pursue a career in biomedical technology. The assistant exclaimed immediately, "That's too bad! Your family's knowledge will be lost!"

Although the three of us understood that Chen had passed along his knowledge to the many students he had trained over the years, nobody objected to the assistant's words. Indeed, we stood there and shared a brief moment of anticipatory nostalgia. Chen was the first to recover, and he assured the assistant that it was not necessary to worry: "My daughter has been copying my prescriptions (*chaofang*) and studying very closely with me. She has always liked Chinese medicine. I'll pass my practice on to her. Besides, a girl's temperament is more suited for Chinese medicine anyway."

I was fascinated by Chen's comments: it was not the first time that I heard practitioners justify passing on their knowledge and practice to daughters rather than sons by the reasoning that women are more suitable to the job. This reasoning runs against an old saying in traditional Chinese medicine "*chuanzi bu chuannü*," which means "pass it on to the son but not the daughter." Indeed, traditional kinship discourses and practices among literati doctors privileged father-son succession over inheritance by daughters. In the absence of a suitable male heir, moreover, daughters-in-law were preferred to daughters on the assumption that daughters would be married out of the family. It is not surprising, then, that practitioners, patients, and anthropologists alike have habitually taken father-son succession to be a patrilineal and patriarchal mode of knowledge transmission in traditional Chinese medicine—that is, a culturally distinctive mode of knowledge reproduction that seems to dissolve and wither in the face of institutionalization, globalization, and encounters with biomedicine.

Between 1939 and 1941 approximately six hundred men and one hundred women were enrolled at the three major academies of traditional Chinese medicine in Shanghai—the "laosanxiao" schools (see the introduction) (Qiu 1998:81). The male to female ratio was six to one. In contrast at SCTCM, and later at SUTCM, the student gender ratio has generally been equal, with the exception of the first three incoming cohorts (1956–1958) where there were significantly more male students (Shi 1997).[5] However, in terms of hiring, hospitals tend to favor male students. Some job advertisements explicitly ask for male candidates. In the San Francisco Bay Area and in California more broadly, although official data of the gender ratio of licensed acupuncturists are not available I estimate that women are in the majority, especially among up-and-coming acupuncturists. For example, the fall 2006 enrollment at the American College of Traditional Chinese Medicine (ACTCM) is 73 percent women (National Center for Educational Statistics 2007), which follows the continuation of a trend since at least the 1990s.

At a quick glance, these stories and statistics seem to reveal a shift in the gender relations of traditional Chinese medicine through the processes of modernization, professionalization, and globalization. There is no question that over the last fifty years women students and practitioners of traditional Chinese medicine have enjoyed increased visibility on both sides of the Pacific. However, the regendering of traditional Chinese medicine is not a simple matter of throwing off the shackles of patriarchy, and it would be premature to proclaim the triumph of gender equity in the discourse and practice of Chinese medicine. A closer look at why women are entering the profession of Chinese medicine complicates any celebratory narrative of gender equity in Chinese medicine today. Why, after all, do practitioners in both Shanghai and the Bay Area repeatedly point out that girls and women are suited for careers in medicine, specifically in traditional Chinese medicine? Over the course of my field research I was given a range of reasons for the gendered career predispositions for Chinese medicine: Girls are careful. Girls are patient. Girls are compassionate. Girls have "natural" affinities with ancient medical literatures (most of which were written by men) that are too much of a bore for restless boys.

These assumptions about family, gender, temperament, and profession are indicative of the complex and ambiguous socialities of kinship and gender at play in the worlding of Chinese medicine. These socialities require a critical analysis of not only the gendering of practitioners and families but also the gendering of knowledges. Such an analysis is my task in this chapter. By investigating the regendering of both families and knowledges of Chinese medicine, I rethink and challenge a set of popular and academic discourses about "patrilineal descent" in the transmission of Chinese medicine—namely that patrilineal and patriarchal kinship marks a distinctive, archaic mode of knowledge production and reproduction in Chinese medicine that will inevitably be made obsolete by the processes of institutionalization, standardization, and globalization.

Thus rather than privileging the experience of male practitioners; I explore how, by negotiating the gendering of families and knowledges, women construct their worlds of knowledges and identities in various relations to family traditions in Chinese medicine. My purpose is to provincialize rather than deny or ignore the role of patriarchy in the production and reproduction of traditional Chinese medicine. By focusing on the minoritized perspectives and experiences of women who enter or leave families of Chinese medicine, I suggest that instead of framed by continuity, progress, and globalization, changing discourses and practices of gender and kinship in Chinese medicine involve the regendering of a hierarchy of knowledges and identities that requires us to pay attention to discontinuity and discordance. I argue that the gendering of knowledges and the gendering of women and families must be considered together in understanding the worlding of traditional Chinese medicine as a set of uneven processes that rely as much on continuity as displacement. To begin, I review some of the ways in which gender and kinship have been represented in popular, medical, and anthropological discourses of traditional Chinese medicine.

Gender and Kinship in and of Traditional Chinese Medicine

In 1989, as an effort to record the clinical expertise and life histories of prominent practitioners and to promote traditional Chinese medicine, the popular health periodical *Shanghai Health and Recovery Magazine* (*Shanghai Kangfu Zazhi*) compiled a volume titled *Biographies of Contemporary Famous (Traditional) Chinese Doctors in Shanghai* (*Shanghai dangdai mingzhongyi liezhuan*). The book includes forty-one short biographies of famous Chinese doctors (*mingzhongyi*) born between 1903 and 1924. According to the editor and the biographers, this group of practitioners collectively represent the generations that played and continue to play instrumental roles in molding the local community of traditional Chinese medicine into its current shape. They did so by participating in the founding of SCTCM in 1956 and setting up its teaching hospitals, as well as by establishing the departments of traditional Chinese medicine in biomedical hospitals. Many of these doctors, in spite of their old age (or rather, as has been argued by Judith Farquhar, because of it), were still active in their day-to-day clinical and educational practices. Some, as I came to learn during my fieldwork, continue to be the most visible champions of traditional Chinese medicine by exerting influence on municipal and national healthcare policies and legislatures, educating the public, and taking part in international exchanges.

The theme of family, notably in terms of the generational practices of traditional Chinese medicine, runs throughout these biographies. Among the forty-one mingzhongyi, twenty-seven grew up in families of three or more generations of practitioners of traditional Chinese medicine, and a few could even trace their family genealogies of traditional Chinese medicine back to the Ming Dynasty (1368–1644). In popular terms they are practitioners of *zuchuan zhongyi,* which literally means "Chinese medicine handed down from family ancestors." In addition, two of the forty-one mingzhongyi come from families of two generations of practitioners; ten do not have any family members from prior generations who practiced traditional Chinese medicine; and two do not specify their family traditions. In sum, over 70 percent of these mingzhongyi grew up in families that handed down their practices from generation to generation. Strikingly, only four women mingzhongyi are included in the forty-one biographies. Furthermore, when tracing family traditions the biographers focus exclusively on the medical practices of male ancestors—fathers, grandfathers, and in some cases uncles (especially paternal uncles).

Together these biographical narratives foreground the instrumental roles of "family"—conceived especially in terms of the father-son succession of family practice—in the production of a mingzhongyi, as well as in the making of knowledges and institutions of traditional Chinese medicine in Shanghai and beyond. Moreover, the emphasis on generational practice, as well as the prestige it holds, makes the antiquity of family lines continuous with the antiquity of traditional Chinese medicine. Such an emphasis on family tradition is unparalleled in the biographies of biomedical practitioners, whether in China or the United States. These biographical discourses, thus, not only represent family tradition as a source of medical prestige and authority in traditional Chinese medicine, but also highlight the centrality of patrilineal descent and patriarchal family in the perpetuation of traditional Chinese medical knowledges and communities. In thus representing the family in and of traditional Chinese medicine, these biographical discourses construct traditional Chinese medicine to be as antique and traditional as it is continuous.

Anthropologists have also observed how vertical lines of descent are often privileged in the deployment of family and kinship in traditional Chinese medicine. Elisabeth Hsu, drawing on her extensive fieldwork in the southwest province of Yunnan, notes that Chinese family ties, especially male bonding, provide the social networks for the secret and personal modes of knowledge transmission that distinguish traditional Chinese medicine from the standardized mode of knowledge transmission in biomedicine. She further observes that while family tradition, especially father-son succession, provides the basis for knowledge and prestige for male practitioners, it systematically excludes women in the family (1999:64). Finally, she suggests that as traditional Chinese medicine becomes institutionalized and scientized these "old ways of learning," which are cemented by the absolute loyalty that a son has for his father (101), are increasingly marginalized by the standardized modes of knowing and learning modeled on biomedicine.

Taken together, the popular, medical, and anthropological discourses have viewed family and kinship as an important and distinctive social institution and practice in traditional Chinese medicine. Chinese kinship is seen as patrilineal and patriarchal in structure and in practice, and kinship ties provide the basis for the knowledge and prestige of male practitioners. Readily accessible to men, these ties serve as the social networks that bind together communities of traditional Chinese medicine. Further, the centrality of kinship in the production of traditional Chinese medical knowledges and communities not only marks the difference between traditional Chinese medicine and biomedicine, but also constructs this difference in terms of traditional and modern, patrilineal and gender inclusive, occult and cosmopolitan. It follows, finally, that the marginalization and perceived dissolution of kinship ties in the production of traditional Chinese medicine is seen as a signal of its transition into the modern world.

The view of patrilineal descent and patriarchal family as a traditional social institution and practice in traditional Chinese medicine has a place within broader anthropological accounts of "kinship-based" production. Kinship-based production is often posited as an earlier developmental stage destined to be replaced by the tributary and then capitalist mode of production. Kinship ties, moreover, are seen as structural barriers to free movement in economy and society (see, e.g., Freedman 1970; Wolf 1982).

This developmental scheme that locates kinship-based production in the "waiting room" of world history, however, has been questioned by a number of anthropologists and historians (Chakrabarty 2000; Pomeranz 2000; Yanagisako 2002). Sylvia Yanagisako in her studies of family silk firms in Como, Italy, argues against the widely held assumption that the family firm is an archaic mode of production linked to Europe's preindustrial past and thus is marginal to modern capitalism. Neither does the Italian family, she argues, mark a culturally distinctive "Italian" capitalism. In paying critical attention to the gender question in kinship, Yanagisako points out that kinship and gender processes, relations, and sentiments are not only sociohistorically constituted but also crucial for the production and reproduction of all forms of capitalism. Gendered sentiments of betrayal, in particular, play instrumental roles in producing new firms and new professional knowledges.

My analysis of "Chinese kinship" and "kinship-based" knowledges and communities in traditional Chinese medicine is inspired by this analytical strategy, especially its emphasis on the sociohistorical situatedness, contingency, and discontinuity as productive forces in kinship and gender processes. I ask, first, how would our understandings of family and kinship practices in Chinese medicine change if we shift our attention to women? As the historian Charlotte Furth (1999) eloquently illustrates, by negotiating the boundaries of gender and class, women healers (and patients) in Chinese history have performed important roles in Chinese medicine that have disrupted the dominance of male practitioners. In particular, a few upper-class women from established medical lineages used family and class prestige to achieve the status of literati doctors. Second, I ask how might our views of the contemporary socialities of Chinese medicine change if we place the gendering of families and knowledges at their center? Finally, as argued by Volker Scheid (2007) in his study of medical lineages and master-disciple relations in Chinese medicine, these relations complement each other, and a shift from the focus on lineage to network may enlarge and enrich our understandings of the ways in which the knowledge of Chinese medicine is transmitted. In light of this, I propose a sideways look at translocal networks—a look at neglected branches and unruly ones— that helps us visualize kinship and gender relations in discontinuous webs rather than linear and continuous treelike forms.

In working through my fieldwork materials, as well as feminist analyses of gender and kinship, I suggest that the singular focus on patrilineal descent can be troubled by the experiences and perspectives of women, especially those who come from families that have practiced traditional Chinese medicine for generations. More importantly, the framing of patrilineal descent as the traditional mode of knowledge and community production locates traditional Chinese medicine in the waiting room of biomedicine, and thus precludes any critical analysis of the ways in which biomedicine and traditional Chinese medicine are mutually constituted through unequal, gendered relations. By looking at Chinese medicine sideways, we might be able to shift our analytical attention to encounters and entanglements and take seriously the work of discontinuity and displacement in translocal formation.

My discussions of the kinship in and of traditional Chinese medicine in this chapter deliberately privilege the ways in which, by becoming traditional Chinese or biomedical practitioners, women experience and negotiate kinship and gender relations in forging their own professional identities. In doing so, I stress the importance of situating the discourses and practices of kinship in and of traditional Chinese medicine within translocal fields where traditional Chinese medicine and biomedicine, tradition and modernity, East and West are produced and held in shifting, gendered relations. I argue that rather than an archaic social institution that marks off the boundary between traditional Chinese medicine and biomedicine, the kinship processes in and of traditional Chinese medicine are shaped by a set of broader, sociohistorically contingent discourses and practices of gender and thereby are reworlded into the present of Chinese medicine.

Specifically, in order to understand a daughter's decision to become a practitioner of either traditional Chinese medicine or biomedicine, I take into account the multiple ways in which traditional Chinese medicine is gendered—not only in terms of gender inequalities within the family tradition and along lines of sex, but also through asymmetrical and sociohistorical processes and especially translocal encounters with biomedicine. I show that, in creatively interpreting and negotiating multiple gender discourses, differently positioned individuals with respect to family tradition in traditional Chinese medicine reinscribe, nudge, and sometimes contest the boundary between traditional Chinese medicine and biomedicine through gendered practices.

The Gendering of Family and Medicine

Some further clarifications of my analytical framing of "gender" and "kinship" are in order here. First, as has been argued by feminist analyses of kinship, labeling Chinese society as characterized by "patrilineal descent" obscures the topic rather than illuminates it (Collier and Yanagisako 1987; Watson 1991; Wolf 1972). Others have pointed out that "Chinese kinship" as an object of anthropological analysis has been an Orientalist production by anthropology itself (Chun 1996). Furthermore, as has been noted by Furth (1999), gender relations in the practice of traditional Chinese medicine have always been contested rather than summarily "patriarchal." Historically, male and female practitioners have long engaged in struggles over medical authority.

Thus rather than assuming "patrilineal descent" or "patriarchal family" to be essential features of Chinese society, I pay special attention to how women position themselves vis-à-vis family traditions in traditional Chinese medicine. Rather than focusing on the practice of father-son succession, I examine the ways in which daughters, especially daughters of male Chinese doctors deemed famous, creatively negotiate their professional, familial, and gender identities by becoming practitioners of traditional Chinese medicine or by choosing the biomedical profession.

In this examination I draw on Bourdieu's distinction between "official kinship" and "practical kinship." In his effort to understand "patrilineal" kinship practices in Algeria, Bourdieu argues that the genealogical tree that the anthropologist constructs is a spatial diagram that can be scanned indifferently from any point in any direction (1977:38). Such a genealogical diagram is a theoretical construct that "merely reproduces the *official* representation of the social structures, a representation produced by application of the structuring principle that is *dominant in a certain respect*, i.e. in certain situations and with a view to certain functions" (34). Yet, the genealogical relationship "is never strong enough on its own to provide a complete determination of the relationship between the individuals it unites" (39–40), and in practice kinship relations are the product of strategies "oriented toward the satisfaction of material and symbolic interests and organized by reference to a determinate set of economic and social conditions" (36). Bourdieu thus points at the rupture between, on the one hand, official kinship ideologies and, on the other, strategic kinship practices that are shaped by positions and interests that in turn are part of broader social structures and cannot be explained by genealogical ties alone. Bourdieu concludes that a close look at how women construct their kinship relations is particularly useful for an analysis of practical kinship, for women's interests and strategies are obscured by the representation of official kinship.

I take from Bourdieu's analysis of practical kinship its emphasis on positionality and situated interests, as well as its insistence that, in order to understand how people actually forge kinship relations, we need to look beyond the conceptual confines of kinship ideologies. Whereas Bourdieu places his analysis of kinship squarely within broader social structure and structured interests that are often explained in utilitarian terms, I am interested in the ways in which gender and kinship relations and practices are shaped by translocal sociohistorical processes, as well as in the partial, multiple, and sometimes mobile positioning of women in relation to these processes.[6] At stake in these relations and practices are a set of personal, professional, and historical identities that go beyond economic or political calculations.

This brings me to my second point about gender. In working within the feminist tradition of kinship and gender analysis, I think of gender not as a distinctive social institution grounded in the "natural fact" of reproductive roles but, as has been argued by Yanagisako and Delaney (1995), as a set of discourses of differentiation that cut across various sites where differences and inequalities are configured—kinship, race, religion, sexuality, nation, modernity. Thus my analysis of gender and kinship not only privileges the experiences of women in the family, but also considers their positioning vis-à-vis broader gendered relations and constructs. In particular I focus on the ways in which women with professional aspirations negotiate their identities by juxtaposing, superimposing, and hence rereading the gendered relations between father and daughter, men and women, biomedicine and traditional Chinese medicine, tradition and modernity, East and West.

In particular I draw on feminist studies of science and medicine. Far from assuming science to be gender neutral or gender inclusive, earlier feminist analyses criticized the exclusion of women from the practice of science and biomedicine (Keller 1983; Rose 1994). Since then, many analysts have extended their critical attention to a wide range of gendered discourses and practices in science and medicine, especially the multiple, discursive ways in which science and biomedicine have come to be masculinized, legitimated, and standardized; for example, by constructing science as a masculine endeavor and nature as a feminine subject (Jordanova 1989; Haraway 1989); by objectifying the female body (Greenhalgh 2001; Haraway 1989; Jordanova 1989; Martin 1992; Rapp 1999); by privileging the masculinist perspective as the only kind of objectivity (Haraway 1991); and by constructing and feminizing Other knowledges (Harding 1998).

It thus follows that we cannot talk about the gendering of traditional Chinese medicine without paying critical attention to the ways in which the discourses and practices of traditional Chinese medicine emerge from its encounters and entanglements with biomedicine. Therefore, rather than reading the perceived marginalization or dissolution of kinship ties—especially father-son succession—in traditional Chinese medicine as signaling the *transition* to modernity, I examine the ways in which discourses of science, modernity, and tradition are *translated* through gendered kinship practices.

In what follows I recount the life stories of three women who came of age in the 1940s when traditional Chinese medicine was in a dire struggle with biomedicine and, incidentally, when patriarchal ideologies also became hegemonic as traditional Chinese medicine took on institutionalized forms. All three women were involved, in different ways, with families of traditional Chinese medicine. Two became practitioners of traditional Chinese medicine, and one became a biomedical practitioner. They were in their late seventies and early eighties at the time of my interviews with them. In other words, they belong to the age group of the mingzhongyi collected in the *Biographies of Contemporary Famous (Traditional) Chinese Doctors in Shanghai*. I chose to talk about this group of women precisely because their experiences and voices are marginalized in the official representation of communities of traditional Chinese medicine. More importantly, in contrasting their radically different life stories and career paths, I emphasize that the kinship and gender in and of traditional Chinese medicine entail positioned, creative, and strategic interpretations and negotiations that produce new forms of uneven socialities even as they reproduce certain old ones.

The Daughter Who Displaced the Son

Dr. Pang Panchi, one of the "miracle workers" discussed in chapter 3, is one of the four women whose lives and careers are included in *Biographies of Contemporary Famous (Traditional) Chinese Doctors in Shanghai.* At the time of our first meeting in 1998, Pang was eighty years old and still active in clinical practices and training students. I first met her at Jiren Clinic, where she worked as a special expert one day a week. She was there at the invitation of Li Fengyi, who had known Pang as a senior colleague at the SUTCM. Li was proud to have her at his clinic, as having one of the most senior and well-respected famous Chinese doctors on staff was a huge boost to the clinic's quality of service and reputation.

Pang's father was a renowned herbalist specializing in internal medicine. Pang studied under her father beginning in her early teens. She also attended the Shanghai College of Traditional Chinese Medicine, a *laosanxiao* school. After her graduation in 1941 she took over her father's clinic, and she practiced there until she was summoned by the government to join Shuguang Hospital in 1954. During our first conversation, I could not help but tell her how excited I was to finally meet a senior female practitioner—everybody else in her age group I had talked to was male. Upon hearing this comment Pang laughed:

> At that time there were professional women in Shanghai, but most of them had teaching and clerical jobs. There were very few doctors. In the beginning, there were a handful of us women [doctors]—no more than three or four—who started around the same time. Girls *had to* be mentored by fathers! In the old days, women were really discriminated against. We could not have gone to school and opened businesses all by ourselves. I studied at the Shanghai College of Traditional Chinese Medicine, but I apprenticed at my father's clinic. He was a famous doctor and had many patients. Little by little, his patients became my patients. Only in this way was I able to eventually hang a sign bearing my own name [*guapai*] in front of the clinic.

According to Pang, if family tradition was considered to be a precious source of knowledge and prestige for boys then it was even more indispensable in the making of a girl's career. Pang's observation is confirmed by information given in *Biographies of Contemporary Famous (Traditional) Chinese Doctors in Shanghai:* whereas twenty-five out of the thirty-seven male practitioners (67.6 percent) had family backgrounds in traditional Chinese medicine, all four female practitioners (100 percent) were from families of traditional Chinese medicine.[7] Thus, even though patriarchal kinship and gender ideologies privileged father-son succession, they did not completely determine a daughter's position within the family or her career path. Ironically, the father's medical knowledge and prestige became an even more important symbolic and cultural capital for the daughter if she were to make a place for herself in the male-dominated profession and in society more broadly. In fact, the father-daughter nexus made it possible for women to enter the profession of traditional Chinese medicine, which was considered masculine relative to the more feminine professions of teaching and clerking that were considered appropriate for middle-class women at the time.

Pang, moreover, was not just any ordinary daughter. She reminisced about a symbolic moment in her life and career: "When I was seventeen or eighteen, the Japanese attacked and took over Pudong. My family escaped to the British Concession in Shanghai.[8] My mother had bound feet, so I did everything—carrying the luggage, buying new furniture and household items . . . Later my father decided to open a clinic in the downtown area. A bunch of hooligans came to our house (where the clinic was located) to ask for 'protection money.' My older brother was very timid. He was so scared that he went and hid inside. It was my uncle (mother's brother) and I who stood at the door and stopped them!"

Pang narrated her gender identity in relation to her mother and older brother. In contrast to her mother, who "had bound feet," Pang was an unmistakably "modern" woman who was fully mobile and able to support the family in times of uncertainty. While her mother's femininity was seen as the product and symbol of tradition and backwardness, Pang subverted this kind of femininity by asserting herself as a modern woman. Moreover, her playful and determined engagement with gender politics did not end there: the comparison between Pang and her older brother was even more striking. While the older brother was "timid" and went *inside* the house when confronted with a situation that required a display of manliness, Pang stood next to her uncle and stopped the hooligans at the door. In so doing Pang took her older brother's place, literally and symbolically. It is noteworthy that Pang organized her narrative around the most recognizable tropes of gender and modernity: mobility and the division of space into outside and inside, public and private. Her displacement of her older brother as their father's heir entailed the switch of gender roles: she presented a masculinized modern daughter and an effeminized son. In other words, even though the daughter displaced the son she did so only by reinscribing the gendered nature of father-son succession, as well as the masculinity of traditional Chinese medicine.

A Grandfather's "American Way of Thinking"

I met Liu Hanchao at her and her husband's house in a suburban town on the peninsula south of the San Francisco Bay. She was in her early eighties at the time of our interview in summer 1999. Having retired from practicing acupuncture only a few years earlier, she and her husband, an engineer, were very involved with their local church.

Liu graduated from the old Shanghai College of Traditional Chinese Medicine in 1940, a year before Pang. After practicing acupuncture in the southwest city of Kunming and then in Shanghai for forty years, she immigrated to the Bay Area in the early 1980s. She then took the California acupuncture licensing exam, obtained a license, and practiced at a friend's clinic until retirement.

Unlike Pang and most other successful female practitioners of her generation, Liu did not have a family background in traditional Chinese medicine. However, she forged a family of traditional Chinese medicine of her own—with the help of her U.S.-educated maternal grandfather. In tracing her career, Liu first told me about her grandfather's encounter with traditional Chinese medicine, an event that shaped her own career:

> My grandfather was educated in the United States. He was among the first group of children, aged between ten and eleven, sent to be educated in the United Stated by the Empress Dowager Cixi. He was in the United States for ten years. After he returned to Shanghai, he was so used to the American way of thinking that he would go to Western doctors exclusively whenever he got sick.
>
> In his old age, perhaps due to high blood pressure, he had severe nose bleeding. When it got really bad, my (maternal) uncle took him to the

Union Medical College Hospital, and he was in the hospital for three days.[9] The Western doctors could not figure out why he was bleeding and suggested surgery. My grandfather got very upset, and said to them, "You can't diagnose the disease, and now you want to open my skull like a watermelon?!"

He got out, and someone introduced him to a traditional Chinese doctor. My mother, his eldest daughter, accompanied him on the visit, and brought a wash basin to catch the blood that kept coming out of his nose. The doctor said to him, "I'll put two [acupuncture] needles in you and you'll be fine." That was exactly what happened. He stopped bleeding and did not need the wash basin anymore! The doctor also gave him an herbal prescription. After taking the herbs for a few days, he was completely cured.

Liu's vivid narrative of her grandfather's "miraculous" cure exemplifies the way in which advocates use "clinical miracles" to demonstrate the clinical efficacy of traditional Chinese medicine, and even its superiority to biomedicine (see chapter 3). What is even more striking in this case is that the grandfather was educated in the United States and, according to Liu, was a practitioner of "the American way of thinking." Moreover, until his problem with nose bleeding, he "would go to Western doctors exclusively whenever he got sick." The beginning part of Liu's narrative thus makes explicit the continuity between her grandfather's "American way of thinking" and his exclusive reliance on biomedicine. In doing so, Liu understood her grandfather's conversion to traditional Chinese medicine as more than a personal experience and decision: she constructed her narrative as a commentary on the relations of East and West, traditional Chinese medicine and biomedicine.

The crux of Liu's commentary is the question of science and rationality—or, to be more exact, the positions of traditional Chinese medicine and biomedicine vis-à-vis science and rationality. According to Liu, the Western doctors not only could not properly diagnose her grandfather's condition, but also exposed their irrationality further by wanting to open his skull "like a watermelon." The U.S.-trained, science-minded grandfather with a bleeding nose was understandably outraged. The narrative's earlier emphasis on the perceived continuity between "the American way of thinking" and biomedicine thus only serves to dramatize their rupture. In contrast, the traditional Chinese doctor, according to Liu, was all about rationality. As she explained: "The Chinese doctor later told me that he needled two acupuncture points on the fingers. These are points along the lung meridian, and the lung meridian opens up [*kaiqiao*] on the nose. So, you see, Chinese medicine is rational and scientific—not a crap shoot!"

In narrating and contrasting her grandfather's clinical encounters with biomedicine and traditional Chinese medicine, Liu reversed the positions of traditional Chinese medicine and biomedicine in relation to science and rationality while still assuming the West to be the referent for science and rationality. Not only did she question the continuity between science and biomedicine, but she also argued for the rationality of traditional Chinese medicine through the intensely personal experience and authoritative affirmation of her grandfather—a United States-trained, science-minded, rational patriarch.

Liu went on to tell me that her grandfather was so enthralled with traditional Chinese medicine that he wanted Liu, his favorite grandchild, to become a disciple (*tudi*) of the Chinese doctor who cured him. As Liu recalled:

> My grandfather was so impressed with this doctor that he wanted him to teach me Chinese medicine, especially acupuncture. The doctor did not want to teach me because it would take a lot of time and energy to train a student. My grandfather had many talks with him. Finally, the doctor gave in. He asked my grandfather to bring me in so that he could see if I was the "right material." We went the next day in the early morning. I don't remember what questions he asked me, but I guess I *was* the "right material" because he agreed to teach me. My mentor [*shifu*] asked for a fee of thirty Chinese silver dollars [*dayang*] a month, and my grandfather was so delighted that he paid him cash on the spot. So, I became his disciple. At the same time, I enrolled at the Shanghai Professional School of Traditional Chinese Medicine. But shifu taught me everything I know about acupuncture.

The word shifu, generally translated as "teacher" or "mentor," literally means "teacher-father." Although in Liu's day most teachers of traditional Chinese medicine were indeed male, today the word shifu is used regardless of the actual gender of the teacher and mentor, and thus it embodies even as it obscures gender and kinship dimensions.[10]

Moreover, between the 1920s and the 1940s it was common practice for students—including those who came from families that had practiced traditional Chinese medicine for generations—to go to one of the three local academies of traditional Chinese medicine while at the same time study and apprentice with their own shifu or fathers (Qiu 1998). These "institutional" and "kinship-based" ways of learning were mutually constitutive rather than exclusive. Many students found their shifu among the faculty at these academies. These institutions in turn supported this kind of mentor-disciple relations: for example, some of the most valued students-disciples went on to join the faculty. Liu's case was unusual—not because she combined "institutional" and "kinship-based" ways of learning, but because her shifu, an acupuncturist, was not a faculty person at any of these institutions.

The practitioners who are Liu's contemporaries wrote or talked about the elaborate rituals of *baishi*—that is, saluting the shifu, which would mark the beginning of a mentor-disciple relationship. The ceremony usually involved a formal salute to the shifu (kowtow, in many cases), a lavish banquet in honor of the shifu and his close friends and colleagues, incense burning for Daoist deities and ancestors of the shifu's family, and a cash present for the shifu. The formality and sumptuousness of the ceremony served to underscore the beginning of an important kinship relation—the memoirs of Liu's contemporaries told stories of how disciples still thought of their shifu's house and family as their own even after starting their own clinic.

These rituals are no longer common practices in Shanghai today. However, the kinship dimension of the mentor-disciple relationship did not simply dissolve—when applying for a master's or doctorate program in traditional Chinese medicine, applicants are required to fill in the name of the practitioner with whom they wish to study. In everyday practice in China, moreover, students of traditional Chinese medicine still refer—sometimes playfully and sometimes emphatically—to their principal advisors as shifu. Classmates, especially those who follow the same principal advisor, are still sometimes referred to as *shixiong* (older brother under the same teacher), *shidi* (younger brother under the same teacher), *shijie* (older sister under the same teacher), and *shimei* (younger sister under the same teacher).

In seeking a shifu then, Liu was able to enter the world of traditional Chinese medicine by forging new kinship ties. Even more interestingly, as her relationship with her shifu's family deepened, she found herself closer to her *shimu* ("teacher-mother"), the wife of her shifu. When the Japanese army invaded Shanghai in 1937, Liu's shifu escaped to the southwest city of Kunming. After he settled down, he wrote back to his wife asking her to join him. Too afraid to go by herself, the wife asked Liu to accompany her. Liu made the trip with her shimu in 1940, even though it meant that she was not able to take part in her graduation commencement at the Shanghai College of Traditional Chinese Medicine. After the journey Liu settled in Kunming. When her shifu passed away soon afterward, she married a local practitioner of traditional Chinese medicine, and they set up their own clinic.

As Liu's career progressed, her ties to her natal family were gradually eclipsed by her involvement with her chosen family of traditional Chinese medicine—first through her physical removal by migration, then through her marriage in which there was little trace of her natal family's presence. In leaving her natal family behind, she played the role of a disciple and daughter by standing by her shimu, especially in the absence of her shifu. In the end, her search for new kinship ties with traditional Chinese medicine was completed by her marriage in Kunming and the subsequent opening of their clinic.

It is noteworthy that in Liu's career and kinship practices she did not simply forsake a modern, cosmopolitan, Western world for a medical practice that was traditional and kinship-based. Indeed, the person responsible for starting her off on her career path was none other than her U.S.-educated grandfather. In other words, it was precisely her grandfather's transnational experiences and his encounters with both biomedicine and traditional Chinese medicine that made it possible for Liu to take the first step in seeking a profession that she—and her grandfather by her account—considered every bit as rational and scientific as biomedicine, if not more so.

The transnational dimension of Liu's career choice was by her account further sharpened through the encouragement she received from her maternal uncle. As she noted: "My maternal uncle was studying in France when I took up Chinese medicine. When he came back, he asked me if the curriculum at the Shanghai College of Traditional Chinese Medicine included acupuncture. I told him that the college taught mostly herbal medicine but not acupuncture, and that I was learning acupuncture from my shifu. My uncle was delighted to hear that I was studying acupuncture. He said, 'The French are all doing acupuncture. How could we Chinese not study acupuncture?!'" As noted earlier, people in China (as well as herbalists elsewhere) largely considered herbal medicine to be the essence of traditional Chinese medicine. For various historical reasons, however, outside of China and especially outside of East Asia acupuncture came to be seen and practiced as the main component of traditional Chinese medicine. For example, the introduction of acupuncture to France was mediated by its colonial ties with Vietnam, where acupuncture was emphasized over herbal medicine (Eckman 1996). Thus the nationalist sentiments of Liu's uncle (as well as Liu's own) regarding traditional Chinese medicine were transnationally produced through the uncle's personal experience in France and through larger colonial processes.

By including this incident as one of the pivotal moments in the early years of her career, Liu made it clear that her own choice of acupuncture over herbal medicine was not about returning to the antique and occult but rather was decidedly transnational. Interestingly, while she obtained her knowledge of herbal medicine through her studies at the college, she learned, in her own words, everything she knew about acupuncture from her shifu. That which was the most antique and occult turned out to be the most cosmopolitan.

It was Liu's grandfather's traveling experiences, as well as his wealth, that made it possible for her to enter a kinship relation with her shifu. Conversely, it was by participating in the seemingly antique, kinship-based mode of knowledge and community production that Liu was able to fulfill her and her grandfather's cosmopolitan visions of science and medicine. The complex, interwoven narrative of Liu's career trajectory and kinship practice moves across and rearranges a set of gendered boundaries—East and West, traditional Chinese medicine and science, tradition and modernity, kinship-based modes of knowledge production and institutional ones, nationalism and transnationalism—even as it reinscribes other more conventional gender roles.

Rebellious Daughters

The last story in the group is really a set of stories. Rather than adding up to a single, larger story, they intersect, loop back, and sometimes contradict each other. The first story in the set is about a family of men.[11] During my fieldwork in Shanghai, apart from interviewing practitioners about their life stories and local history of medicine, I also made it my task to read through the memoirs and biographies of senior practitioners, as well as the official histories of the local institutions and communities of traditional Chinese medicine. With almost no exception, when reading these memoirs, biographies, and histories I would come across members of the Dong family. These texts focused mostly on Dong Yixin, his second son Dong

Zhongda, his grandson Dong Runhua (the eldest son of Dong Yixin's eldest son), and the male disciples of the family (many of whom were the authors of the memoirs, biographies, and histories that I read). Dong Yixin was born two decades after the First Opium War, and his career peaked in the 1910s and 1920s. Zhongda and Runhua—the former born before and the latter born after the turn of the twentieth century—were most active in the 1930s and 1940s.

Dong Yixin, the patriarch, was one of the most celebrated practitioners of traditional Chinese medicine in Shanghai, and he himself came from a prestigious lineage of practitioners. He was remembered for organizing and leading the practitioners in Shanghai in their struggles with biomedicine and with the republic government's campaigns against traditional Chinese medicine. Dong became one of the founding fathers of the Shanghai Professional School of Traditional Chinese Medicine in 1916, and it was at this school that he trained a large group of male students who themselves went on to become highly successful practitioners, educators, and, in some cases, activists. These students—including Dong's male offspring and disciples—not only continued their teacher's intellectual legacy, but also played instrumental roles in the institutionalization of traditional Chinese medicine by holding top administrative and teaching positions upon the founding of SCTCM in 1956.

Dong Yixin's firstborn son died young, leaving both Runhua and his uncle Zhongda to be closely mentored by Yixin. Both were able to observe and learn from his daily clinical practice, as well as study under other teachers at the Shanghai Professional School of Traditional Chinese Medicine where they were students.[12] Both Runhua and Zhongda became highly accomplished and well-respected practitioners, educators, and activists in their own right. Yet kinship ideologies and practices among the literati class favored primogeniture. Moreover, as suggested by the memoir of one of Dong Runhua's disciples, the untimely death of Runhua's father made Yixin dote even more on the grandson. Thus it was Runhua who inherited the family mansion, the primary family clinic housed in the mansion, and Yixin's leadership positions at the school and at local professional organizations. Zhongda, on the other hand, inherited the family's secondary clinic, which was bought by Yixin. Runhua and Zhongda both moved to Hong Kong shortly before 1949, and Runhua passed away in the mid-1960s. Zhongda immigrated to the United States in the early 1950s, and he lived in the San Francisco Bay Area until he passed away almost thirty years later.

The Dong mansion was more than just a family house and clinic. During my interview with Lu Hanqiu, a senior practitioner who was a disciple of Dong Runhua's, he described the mansion as it was during the Dong family's heyday in the late 1930s:

> I graduated from the Shanghai College of Traditional Chinese Medicine in 1942. My shifu was Dong Runhua. . . . His house was an old-fashioned Chinese house in the British Concession. My *taishifu* ["grandfather-teacher" Dong Yixin] bought it. There were more than fifty rooms in that house. Shifu's clinic took up two rooms on the second floor. There was a part of the house that was more like a dorm—many students who studied at the school lived there and learned medicine.
>
> My shifu used to receive more than one hundred patients a day and pay up to twenty house calls in the evening. I followed him around. He did not have any time to do any writing. He wouldn't be back home until 2:00 in the morning. Then he would sit down and eat, and would invite me to eat at the same table. But I would be too exhausted to eat anything. I don't know how he was able to manage it—his students rotated shifts, but he had to work everyday.

The activities in the Dong mansion were also described in similar ways in the memoirs of other disciples of the family. The Dong mansion in Runhua's day thus included within its boundary his family, students, and patients—in other words, his clinical, educational, institutional, and familial practices. By including them within the bounds of his household, Dong Runhua nurtured the next generation of traditional Chinese medicine.

Moreover, Lu had a more special personal relationship with Runhua than did many of his other disciples. As he noted: "Shifu was especially nice to me. He had a son who was my classmate. We used to sit next to each other in class. A lot of people said that we looked alike. This son died very young. So, I think when shifu saw me, I reminded him of his dead son." Lu, who was well into his seventies at the time of our conversation, never forgot to reciprocate the attention that his teacher and father bestowed on him. He told me that he accomplished three feats for his shifu: compiling a who's who volume of the students attending the school between 1917 and 1948; writing a volume on Dong Runhua's scholarly thoughts; and helping to edit the history of the laosanxiao schools.

Taken together, Lu, as well as the authors of the memoirs, biographies, and local history texts, accentuated the solidarity of the local communities of traditional Chinese medicine in their accounts of the Dong family. This solidarity was produced through encounters and struggles with biomedicine, and it was mediated by the construction of kinship ties that brought together families and institutions, individuals and communities. For many, solidarity with the Dong family was the solidarity of the local communities. Lu, for example, saw his efforts in compiling the local history of traditional Chinese medicine as a tribute to his teacher Dong Runhua. The story of the Dong family was thus an integral part of the story of traditional Chinese medicine in Shanghai. And, as it was told, it was also a story of men.

None of the memoirs, biographies, and history texts made any reference to the lives and careers of women in the Dong family. The only context in which women appeared under their birth names was in the chronology of male family members' marriages and births, where a woman was acknowledged as a wife, concubine, or mother. No daughters were mentioned. In one biography it was noted that Dong Runhua's wife was the daughter of another famous practitioner, and her marriage to Runhua solidified the kinship bonds between the two families of (male) practitioners.

The absence of women in these memoirs, biographies, and history texts left me with the initial impression that, other than serving their reproductive and domestic roles, the women in the family did little worth mentioning—at least not in the context of the history of traditional Chinese medicine. I could not have been more wrong in this view, however. In what follows I recount the second story of the Dong family.

The story begins with my meeting with Dr. Hsiang Tung, M.D. It was toward the end of my fieldwork in the San Francisco Bay Area that I met Hsiang at the apartment that she and her husband owned in an upscale suburban neighborhood. Prior to our meeting, the only information I had about her was that she was a biomedical doctor who had lent much support to the American Foundation of Traditional Chinese Medicine in its early days. After retirement from her position at a hospital in the Midwest in the mid-1980s, Hsiang decided to settle down in the Bay Area.

Unlike my interviews with Pang and Liu, my interview with Hsiang was conducted largely in English. I began the conversation by telling her briefly about my research on traditional Chinese medicine. In response, she said that she had just attended a qigong class taught by two Chinese students at Stanford University. She said that one of her friends who went with her claimed to feel much better when doing the exercise. She didn't elaborate, so I asked her how she felt about it. Laughing, she replied: "I'm not sure what I got out of it—I'm not a Buddhist. They were talking about 'cultivating qi,' and that you'd go up different levels to achieve some kind of Buddhist awareness. I'm a Christian. I'm not sure how the levitation could happen."

Recalling that the American Foundation of Traditional Chinese Medicine's current project was introducing elementary school students in the San Francisco Unified School District to the practice of qigong (albeit a rudimentary form), I made the decision to change the topic. I asked Hsiang how she became involved with traditional Chinese medicine. She said it was because a former colleague of hers became interested and encouraged her to learn acupuncture after retirement. She went to Shanghai in the 1980s and learned acupuncture at Shuguang Hospital. She never practiced acupuncture in the United States, however, even though as a medical doctor she was legally eligible to do so. It was relatively easy for her to study acupuncture in Shanghai because she still had some distant relatives there; in fact, her own father was an herbal doctor in Shanghai. These family relations came almost as an afterthought to Hsiang. But I persisted:

"What's his name?"

"Dong Runhua."

This was one of the most surprising revelations during my fieldwork, and the story that ensued was among the most fascinating ones I encountered. As Hsiang told me: "I know from my father that if you want to learn Chinese medicine, you have to start very young. My father had ten children. I was the firstborn. Two younger brothers were traditional Chinese medicine practitioners. They started with my father when they were twelve or thirteen. Another one was a Ph.D. in genetic engineering. Another brother went to Japan to learn acupuncture. Then he came to the U.S. the same year when James Reston got his acupuncture [1971].[13] He was very busy in New York—seeing patients and taking part in legalizing acupuncture. He passed away a few years ago."

Two of Dong Runhua's sons continued their father's practice in herbal medicine. A third one took a more transnational career trajectory by studying acupuncture and physiotherapy in Japan, and then taking part in the efforts to legalize acupuncture in New York. Indeed, he was one of the most outspoken champions of acupuncture and traditional Chinese medicine in the early 1970s: he was arrested for practicing medicine without a license, and his high-profile court case helped raise public awareness of acupuncture on the East Coast.[14] Thus as the history of traditional Chinese medicine in the United States also became entangled with the family history of the Dongs, the Dong family's legacy in traditional Chinese medicine continued.

The daughters of the family, in contrast, made radically different career choices. Hsiang herself was one of the three biomedical doctors in the family—the other two included a daughter of Dong Yixin's and a daughter of Dong Zhongda's. Hsiang told me about their stories:

> I didn't go into Chinese medicine because I went to Zhongxi Girls' School [in Shanghai], a missionary school.[15] I came to the U.S. after high school. That was in 1941. I went to Mount Holyoke for undergraduate education. Then I went to the University of Michigan for medical school. My grandaunt helped me get a scholarship for medical school. Nobody in my family objected to my studying Western medicine. They were Buddhists and I'm a Christian. They were very open. . . .
>
> Speaking of my grandaunt [a daughter of Dong Yixin's]: she was a renegade! Her family forced her to marry a man that she did not think deserving of her. She was also at Zhongxi Girls' High School at the time. Her teachers helped her run off to America. So she ran away—three days before the wedding. Her family had already prepared the banquet! She went to Mount Holyoke, studied medicine, and became a gynecologist. She later went back to Tianjin [a northern city in China], and opened her own hospital. She never got married, and dedicated her whole life to medicine. She was a very strong person.
>
> My granduncle's daughter [Dong Zhongda's daughter] was also a Western doctor. My grandaunt helped her [with her career] as well.

I was fascinated by the stories of the daughters of the Dong family, especially Dong Yixin's daughter. The events in her life were extraordinary in their own terms, which made even more striking the complete silence with regard to her life and career in the written histories of the Dong family. I could only speculate that the disciples who compiled those histories considered her career and life choice a scandal, if not a betrayal. Dong Yixin's daughter was indeed a "renegade": she constructed her own familial and professional identity by subverting hegemonic, patriarchal gender and kinship relations. She defied her role as a daughter by ditching the wedding arranged for her by her family; she escaped all the way across the Pacific to the United States. She chose biomedicine, and she went back to China to set up a biomedical hospital. To top it off, she reconfigured the gender and professional alignment of her familial ties by helping other daughters of the family into careers in biomedicine in the United States. It bears mentioning, further, that all of this happened at a time when the men in her family were struggling to ensure the survival of traditional Chinese medicine. It is remarkable, then, that by the time Hsiang decided to go abroad to study biomedicine, there was, she states, no objection from her family.

Thus it is not surprising that the career and life choices of the daughters of the Dong family were extraordinary not only for the family but also for the larger communities of traditional Chinese medicine in Shanghai. The histories of the Dong family and the larger communities, as they were written and narrated by male practitioners, were narratives of inclusion and solidarity grounded in bonds between men and forged in opposition to biomedicine. These daughters were out of place—by being women and by being biomedical practitioners. The case of Dong Yixin's daughter in particular shows that while the patriarchal ideologies provided the ground for inclusive kinship practices and the production of the knowledges and communities among men, the same ideologies and practices drove a woman away from her family and traditional Chinese medicine. As Hsiang put it, "It seems like all the men in my family went for the East, and the women went for Western medicine!"

By contrasting "the East" to "Western medicine" rather than "the West," Hsiang's remarks accentuated the relational production of places, knowledges, and identities. "The East" was not a discrete, value-neutral geographical locale; neither was "Western medicine" a freestanding medical system and practice. Rather, Hsiang's commentary highlighted a set of gendered place- and identity-making strategies that superimposed kinship processes with translocal encounters and networks of knowledges and communities. The daughters of the Dong family invoked and appropriated a set of translocal, gendered relations—East and West, traditional Chinese medicine and biomedicine—in subverting patriarchal kinship ideologies and practices at home. Thus in Hsiang's commentary "the East" and "Western medicine" already embodied multiple, intersecting, and at times contradictory gender processes. It follows then, that the gendering of women and men, East and West, traditional Chinese medicine and biomedicine was not defined by fixed structural oppositions; instead, it was precisely through gendered traveling routes and practices that these differences and asymmetries were produced, negotiated, and transformed.[16]

The gendered relations between biomedicine and traditional Chinese medicine and between father and daughter were further underscored in Hsiang's comments about her father's clinical practice:

> After I came to the U.S., there was Pearl Harbor. I did not hear from my parents again until 1946. My father had a lot of patients, including Kuomintang VIPs. So when the communists came, he moved to Hong Kong. After I finished my internship and residency, my daughter was already five years old. We went to visit my family in Hong Kong. That was 1955.
>
> When I was there, there was a child who had a huge, egg-size growth underneath one side of his chin. It was probably an abscess or a swollen lymph node. I called all the pediatricians in town and nobody was available. So I called my dad. We took the child to see him. He gave him some herbs to apply externally, and some herbal tea to drink. And, I was *shocked* to find that the swelling was absorbed the next day. Normally, with Western medicine, we would probably have to open the abscess and drain it, and then use penicillin and other antibiotics. So, I thought, my dad really is something!

In narrating this incident, Hsiang positioned herself not only as a daughter but also as a biomedical practitioner. In this sense Dong Runhua produced double "miracles": he accomplished, at one level, what biomedicine could not do; at the same time he was able to get the job done when his daughter and her pediatrician colleagues failed to deliver. Strikingly, even though by 1955 Dong Runhua was already a highly accomplished practitioner of traditional Chinese medicine, it was only when Hsiang witnessed his clinical success in relation to her own failure that she came to the conclusion that he "really is something." Hsiang's "approval" of her father thus was subversive of the hegemonic gender and kinship relations between father and daughter, and the approval came by appropriating and reaffirming biomedicine as the masculinist, authoritative referent for clinical efficacy.

Hsiang's strategic positioning as a masculinist biomedical practitioner came out even more sharply in her interpretation of the significance of this incident—or what she called an "anecdote." As she went on to tell me, "I think Chinese medicine needs to be more scientific. My colleagues in traditional Chinese medicine all have a lot of anecdotes, but no statistics." Thus, even though her father might have impressed her, Hsiang's approval did not extend to traditional Chinese medicine overall. Indeed, if anything the event only underscored what she saw as the anecdotal nature of clinical success in traditional Chinese medicine.

In contrast to the neat, chronologically organized display at the Museum of the History of Traditional Chinese Medicine, following the narratives of family and gender does not lead us back to a point of origin of traditional Chinese medicine but instead opens up and entangles us in a shifting network of people, ideas, institutions, and histories that are open to rewriting and rethinking. In telling the stories of these three women and their families, I do not intend to fit narratives by the men and women of traditional Chinese medicine together into a coherent, comprehensive history and panoramic view. They do not constitute "women's experience" or "women's perspective" that would complete an existing story. Rather, these stories foreground discontinuities and diverging trajectories in the worlding of Chinese medicine. On the one hand, the memoirs, biographies, and history texts written by male disciples and descendants celebrate the solidarity, continuity, and resilience of local and translocal communities of Chinese medicine, as well as the masculinity of Chinese medicine. Alternately, the life stories and career trajectories of the women of families of traditional Chinese medicine can be read as productions of a set of translocal, gendered connectivities that not only problematize the masculine discourses of Chinese medicine and Chinese kinship, but also bring to the fore the gendered relations between Chinese medicine and biomedicine, East and West. My strategy, then, has been to hold in tension the multiple, intertwined, and sometimes contradictory and discontinuous socialities of gender and kinship at play in the worlding of Chinese medicine. In presenting the narratives of the life stories and career trajectories of Pang, Liu, and the daughters of the Dong family, I have privileged women's experiences and strategies to foreground the ways in which their lives and careers—as well as their understandings of them—are always already positioned in relation to tropes of the family that are inextricable from gendered sociohistorical processes. These processes configure and translate East and West, tradition and modernity, traditional Chinese medicine and biomedicine, miracle and science.

Furthermore, discourses of kinship and gender provide a contingent ground for differently situated people to negotiate and reconfigure specific forms of knowledges and identities, and to forge particular kinds of connections and alliances. This kind of approach helps us understand the socialities of gender and kinship in and of traditional Chinese medicine today. For example, instead of interpreting a father's decision to pass on his trade to the daughter simply as the triumph of the struggle for gender equality, we need to also consider how traditional Chinese medicine is feminized in relation to biomedicine. By the same logic, rather than understanding a son's decision to become a biomedical practitioner as the dissolution of the traditional mode of father-son succession, we may see it as a way of renegotiating the boundary of traditional Chinese medicine and biomedicine by including the latter within the hegemonic "family tradition." An examination of kinship and gender both vertically and sideways highlights processes of both connection and displacement, making and unmaking. Far from an archaic mode of knowledge production and transmission, gendered family ties—stretching tenuously both vertically and sideways, through thick and thin—reach deep into the present and future of traditional Chinese medicine.

Six

DISCREPANT
DISTANCES

As the first decade of the new millennium draws toward an end, it has become all too easy to talk about the aspiration and ascendance of China as a global economic and political power—an ascendance staged against the precarious position of the United States as the world's only superpower. Indeed, it would seem strange not to pay attention to the increasing global visibility of China. Breathtaking phrases such as "the Chinese century" and "China rising" have made headlines in popular magazines, newspapers, and television programs in the United States (Elliot 2007; Fishman 2004). In casual conversations my friends in California sometimes ask me, "Has China taken over yet?" Even the near 10 percent fall of the Shanghai and Shenzhen stock markets just after the Lunar New Year on February 28, 2007, which sent shock waves through the American, European, and Asian markets, was read by many in the United States and China alike as an indication of China's new global prominence.[1]

Shanghai, China's "crown jewel" (Heim 2001), figures centrally in this story of ascendance: the *China Rises* television series, cosponsored by the *New York Times* and the Discovery Times Channel, focuses one of its four episodes entirely on Shanghai as a city that is "culturally cutting-edge" and "forward looking." These sentiments are perhaps most acutely felt in the city of Shanghai itself. In a volume on the *haipai* (Shanghai-style) lifestyle, Li Haoran writes, "When we walk past big shopping malls such as Plaza 66, the CITIC building, Printemps, and Isetan,[2] city dwellers of Shanghai really feel that the time lag and distance between us and world-famous brand-name commodities is zero. Does this mean that the distance between the vicinities of Pudong, Huaihai Road, and Nanjing Road and the elegance of Champs Elysées and Fifth Avenue is zero? And so close to the class and taste of the Elizabeth Hurleys, the Cindy Crawfords, and the Claudia Schiffers that there is no 'jet lag' at all?" (2006:225). The imminence of a "Chinese century" spearheaded by Shanghai, however, would have been hard to imagine a mere decade ago. As a taxi took me out of the Hongqiao International Airport when I arrived for my fieldwork in Shanghai on a July evening in 1998, I was struck by an eerie feeling at the sight of row after row of unoccupied, unlit office and residential buildings—some brand new and others at various stages of construction—that lined the darkened streets. It was the height of the so-called Asian economic crisis.[3] Shanghai, though largely unscathed, was gripped by an overwhelming sense of anxiety: "Have we overdeveloped? What if we built the house and no one came?" The future seemed anything but certain: even though the slogan "get on track with the world" was all the rage, there were murmurs that it was by being *not quite* on track with the world that China, and Shanghai in particular, had evaded the full brunt of the economic crisis. China seemed at once lagging behind *and* having perhaps moved too fast and too far ahead.

In this chapter I try to recapture the ambiguities in translocal spatiotemporal imaginaries by turning my attention to the ways in which "China" is imagined and located through the worlding of traditional Chinese medicine. I discussed in chapter 1 how particular worlds are made, whether in the image of a cosmopolitan, middle-class California or an international proletariat. I suggested that, far from being transcendent, these emergent worlds are deeply entangled in the production of difference. In this chapter I further explore the translocality of the ways in which contingent terms of difference are produced and deployed through the worlding of Chinese medicine. Specifically, by examining the tenuous and contested links between "China," "Chinese culture," and "Chinese medicine," I emphasize that, instead of producing a uniform and ever-expanding global network and community of traditional Chinese medicine, translocal encounters provide occasions for making strategic alliances at the same time that they refashion persisting discourses of difference and create new spatiotemporal disjunctures and disparities. In other words, I suggest that the worlding of Chinese medicine is as much about strategies of distancing and alienation as it is about forging bonds and negotiating commonalities: even though imaginaries of "America" seem readily available and even intimate in the everyday discourse and practice of Chinese medicine in Shanghai, for many practitioners in California "China" remains a shifting, ambiguous sign that is at once close and unreachable, familiar and alien, backward and whirled forward off course.

From Empires to Disparate Connectivity

Until recently, it was popular among the academic left to fashion narratives of "empire" by proclaiming that imperialism was over, and that we had now entered a new global era defined by deterritorialized power. Even though these hypermasculine narratives of empire more or less imploded after September 11, 2001, fascinations with tropes of flow, circulation, and dispersal have continued to shape our analytical habits and possibilities. Although the tropes of flow, circulation, and dispersal have been instrumental in conceptualizing transnationalism and globalization, it is noteworthy that these words have a genealogy in which they are commonly used as apt descriptions of how capital and commodity move. As theories of globalization (e.g., Harvey 1989; Jameson 1988; Sassen 1991) build on—even as they depart from—the political economy of the world-system (Wallerstein 1974; Wolf 1982), they have retained the descriptions of the movements of capital and commodity by renewing and applying them, metaphorically at least, to the analyses of global structures and processes. Having shed some of their genealogical specificities, these tropes have in fact become magnified to cover a plethora of phenomena ranging from migration, development, trade, mass media, science, information technology, and various other forms of cultural production that transgress or exceed the boundaries of the territorially bound nation-state. More important, the focus on circulation, flow, and dispersal has mediated the popular and academic discussions of globalization that locate America, and the West by extension, at the very center of our understandings of the workings of globalization. However, in spite of their popularity and centrality in the discourses of globalization, these tropes do not capture the entire gamut of the ways in which translocal formations take place, nor do they capture the effervescence of translocal socialities. The concept of "circulation" seems too seamless to convey the grittiness and contradictions of the workings of power, while leaving the disparate and the unexpected socialities out of critical analyses. At the same time, "flow" or "dispersal" does not by itself account for the "stickiness"—to use Anna Tsing's word (2005)—of translocal encounters or the role of displacement and breakage in translocal formation. It is with these concerns in mind that I explore other analytics that do not rely on metaphors of how capital and commodity move, and that allow us to think about historicity, heterogeneity, incongruence, ruptures, and practices of location in translocal social formation.

In understanding the production of "America" in particular, a focus on "transnational connectivity," as proposed by Inderpal Grewal (2005:22), offers a tremendously useful analytical alternative. The notion of "transnational connectivity" highlights fields of power where varying degrees and great varieties of connections always exist. In Grewal's work critical attentiveness to connectivity has enabled an important reconsideration of the ways in which "America" is imagined and produced both inside and, perhaps more importantly, outside of the borders of the United States. Instead of assuming the United States to be an imperialist empire that rules through economic and political domination, Grewal argues that America works as an imaginary of neoliberalism that is both consumed and reproduced among South Asian communities inside and outside the United States. Her analysis thus questions the artificial boundaries dividing empires, nation-states, and diasporas—boundaries that rest upon the assumption that these are entirely different zones and scales or incommensurable modes of sociality. To borrow from Engseng Ho (2004), I think that Grewal has shown us how to see the production of the American empire "through diasporic eyes." In other words, she demonstrates the usefulness of methodologies developed in critical feminist diasporic studies to bear on studies of empires and nation-states by foregrounding how they are produced by differentiated imaginaries of scale.

Like Grewal, I am interested in the production of cultural imaginaries through translocal fields of power, in particular, how "America"—as well as "China"—is made through disparate connectivities rather than an empire or nation-state that simply moves up (and down) the global hierarchy of powers. Whereas Grewal discusses how the idea of "America" is fashioned by the Others within and, more important, outside of the border of the United States, I focus here on how differently positioned people remake the imaginaries of the Others—through discussions of culture, tradition, knowledge, science, and politics—in the United States where particular translocal encounters take place. In this chapter I focus on ethnographic encounters in the San Francisco Bay Area in light of how "China," Chinese culture," and "Chinese medicine" are imagined, understood, and invoked by people from varied sociohistorical locations and within particular settings. In particular, I show that conceptions of "culture," "tradition," "science," and "traditional Chinese medicine" are neither assumed nor ignored but rather negotiated and contested in relation to one another. These negotiations and contestations take place through specific translocal routes and discrepant translocal alliances. Whereas Chinese diplomats at international conferences and other gatherings in San Francisco often speak of traditional Chinese medicine as a "bridge of friendship" between East and West upon which one can readily walk, I would instead argue to the contrary. East and West, China and America, and past and future are not fixed and easily identifiable nodes within circuits of globalization but rather are shifting and uneven spatiotemporal imaginaries produced and refigured through particular translocal encounters that are as much about movement and circulation as about displacements and ruptures.

Uncanny Alliances

While conducting research in the San Francisco Bay Area I attended a number of the international conferences on traditional Chinese medicine regularly held in the Bay Area. Organized by local organizations and advocates of traditional Chinese medicine, some of these "global" or "multilateral" conferences, as they are called, are celebratory in nature. Others, however, provide occasions for exchanging clinical knowledge, theoretical papers, and laboratory research results, as well as articulating visions of the future of Chinese medicine.

Key participants in these conferences include practitioners from the Bay Area and from China. Appearances by U.S. politicians, Chinese diplomats, research scientists, professional fundraisers, and various dignitaries are also much sought after by conference organizers. This attraction is not unilateral; for example, local politicians have sought out these conferences as part of their district- and city-level election campaigns. I am not certain how the voters are affected by the visits, but conference participants from China—though generally impressed by appearances by the mayor and by congress members—sometimes look at the politicians with unadulterated perplexity: Why are they here if they do not know anything about Chinese medicine?

In addition, practitioners and advocates of traditional Chinese medicine from Japan, Taiwan, Mexico, and Europe are also drawn to these conferences. They each carry their own versions and professional associations of "traditional Chinese medicine," which as in the United States is referred to by a variety of names, ranging from traditional Chinese medicine, to Oriental medicine, to simply acupuncture.[4] Interestingly, although many African countries played central roles in the worlding of traditional Chinese medicine in the 1960s and the early 1970s, I have yet to see any representatives from Africa at these conferences. On a few occasions I asked the conference organizers about the absence of acupuncturists from Africa. Some replied diplomatically that it would be an interesting idea for future conferences. Others, apparently unaware of the recent activities of Chinese medical entrepreneurs in Africa, pointed out that their conferences were organized to represent the *current* state of traditional Chinese medicine around the world and thus focused on places where acupuncture and herbal medicine were prospering.

To be sure, Africa is not entirely forgotten: in a celebratory speech a Chinese diplomat once made a brief comment about "African countries." In reviewing the history of traditional Chinese medicine, he counted Africa—*before* Japan, the United States, and Europe—among the countries and areas reached by traditional Chinese medicine. As indicated by this diplomat's remarks and by the absence of representatives from Africa at these "global" conferences, the place of Africa in the worlding of traditional Chinese medicine has been for the most part relegated to "history."

Given the fact that the participants come from a wide array of backgrounds, the broad range of speakers and speeches at these conferences never fails to intrigue me. There are usually four groups of people: senior practitioners who participated in the legalization and mainstreaming of Chinese medicine in the 1970s, younger practitioners in their thirties and forties who currently hold administrative positions in the communities of traditional Chinese medicine in California, international visitors from China and other countries, and Chinese and American government officials who usually make brief appearances either at the beginning of the conference or in the middle of it depending on the schedule of these officials.

In their speeches the senior Californian practitioners and activists— mostly Chinese immigrants but also a few Caucasian Americans—reminisce about the field's early days, especially in the 1970s and the early

1980s. Even though their narratives and opinions differ about who contributed exactly what, they all emphasize that they once literally had to "bang on the doors" of mainstream society in order for acupuncture to be recognized as a legitimate medical practice.

Many of the younger Californian practitioners who attend these conferences currently hold (or aspire to hold) administrative positions in various Californian professional organizations, or else serve on the California Acupuncture Committee—a subdivision of the Department of Consumer Affairs. Compared to the senior practitioners and activists, there is a smaller contingency of Chinese Americans in this younger group, some of whom are native born and locally trained while others are recent immigrants who obtained their medical training in China. In the latter group most are graduates of colleges of traditional Chinese medicine in China; some, however, are students at biomedical universities and have taken acupuncture courses before immigrating to the United States. Although some of these biomedically trained practitioners once intended to go back to biomedicine upon reaching the shores of California, they find it too time consuming and too costly to pass all of the requirements to become an M.D. in the United States.

The speeches by the younger participants tend to focus on the current state of Chinese medicine in California and in the United States more broadly. Their topics regularly include the development of the educational system, licensing practices, legislatures, integration into the medical mainstream, and international exchange. Some of these younger practitioners use interpreters to translate their speeches into Chinese.

Practitioners flying in from China, on the other hand, are for the most part those in important administrative and teaching positions in institutions of traditional Chinese medicine or those who are professionally acclaimed. When talking about traditional Chinese medicine, they often stress both the longevity of the tradition and the importance of its modernization, scientization, and globalization—all of which is consistent with the institutional development of traditional Chinese medicine in China.

Chinese diplomats, perhaps more emphatically than anyone else, structure their speeches around traditional Chinese medicine as a treasure of Chinese culture and civilization, and as a bridge of friendship between China and the United States. They reaffirm that traditional Chinese medicine as a Chinese treasure should be shared by the people of the world. Politicians from the United States who express similar sentiments do so with deliberate ambivalence: the post–cold war period saw extremely fraught geopolitical relations between the People's Republic of China and the United States of America, and it was marked by a series of diplomatic crises on the political, military, and economic fronts. Thus rather than focusing on "the bridge of friendship" the U.S. politicians spend more time in their speeches vouching for their desires to further integrate acupuncture into the medical mainstream in California and in the United States more broadly—a statement that is appealing to local practitioners and activists.

In bringing together speakers and speeches from various historical, social, political, and professional locations, these "global" conferences cast the spotlight on intense moments of translocal encounters. Most strikingly, these conferences, though global or international in name, do not project the image of a growing, uniform global community of Chinese medicine. The bits and pieces do not add up to a panorama. What these global conferences do epitomize, however, are the multiple, intersecting, sometimes diverging trajectories of traditional Chinese medicine, as well as the sociohistorical contingency and situatedness of the translocal actor-networks through which traditional Chinese medicine is worlded.

As I discussed in the previous chapters, emerging from the translocal movement and reconfiguration of traditional Chinese medicine is not a uniform global space promising to transcend particular cultural imaginaries. The fact that California—as well as many other places in East Asia, North America, and Europe—is now an important constituency in the translocal trajectories of traditional Chinese medicine does not mean that "China" or "Chinese culture" is merging into an evolving global conglomeration. Neither does "China" or "Chinese culture" readily function as the distant "home" to the global circulation of traditional Chinese medicine.

One of my most memorable moments at global conferences on traditional Chinese medicine came in San Francisco in 2000 when I met a group of practitioners from Shanghai. Among the group was Dr. Xu Qing, one of my teachers at the Shanghai University of Traditional Chinese Medicine (SUTCM) who was always generous with her time and insights. Between speeches we were able to steal away for a few minutes to catch up with each other. Xu told me with great pride that SUTCM had recently received an award for superior educational quality from the Chinese State Department of Education—an honor that neither of the two biomedical universities in Shanghai was able to claim. When I asked who else had come with her to the conference, she looked around and pointed out a few of her companions to me. In addition, she noted, another group of acupuncturists from China had planned to attend the conference, but in the end they could not because they were denied visas by the U.S. consulate in Shanghai.

Dr. Xu went on to say that she was excited to see that so many Americans—from all walks of life—were interested in acupuncture. However, she found it difficult to make Americans truly understand traditional Chinese medicine because they did not have the same cultural environment, and even the "Chinese" in America were not "authentic" (*zhengzong*) anymore.[5] Xu then stated, "In China, everybody knows something about traditional Chinese medicine. We eat different vegetables during different seasons. The Americans eat ice cream all year long. Some people here think of traditional Chinese medicine simply as a therapeutic practice—as acupuncture. I am worried that the bigger, comprehensive picture of traditional Chinese medicine will be lost little by little. Even I myself, after almost twenty years of practice, still feel like I don't fully understand the essence of Chinese medicine. And not being part of Chinese culture certainly would not help understanding Chinese medicine as a whole."[6] I asked Xu whether the conference gave her any new ideas about the future of traditional Chinese medicine. She replied, "We have to do scientific research. Our colleges need to be more like comprehensive universities—Fudan University, for example. Our students will have to strengthen their training in life sciences, in molecular biology."

As Dr. Xu noted in her remarks, the key to learning and practicing "authentic" Chinese medicine was total immersion in "Chinese culture." She considered China to be the natural home of Chinese culture, and it made little difference that she lived in Shanghai—a city known for its haipai reputation. Xu did not hesitate to contrast the yearlong consumption of ice cream by Americans with the Chinese practice of eating seasonal food. However, even though Dr. Xu might not be completely familiar with the eating habits of Americans (and especially Californians), she must have been very aware of the fact that in Shanghai the availability and consumption of many common vegetables were no longer seasonal thanks to hothouses and supermarkets. She must have seen, as I did, youngsters walking down the streets with ice cream cones in their hands even during the freezing days of January.

What, then, compelled her to make such a polarized and almost deliberately simplistic distinction between the American and the Chinese ways of life? I suggest that in order to understand why Dr. Xu constructed the sharp contrast between the Chinese and the Americans, and between Chinese and American cultures, we need to take into consideration the specific settings in which her words were articulated. Having taught and practiced traditional Chinese medicine in Shanghai for nearly twenty years, Xu was all too familiar with the day-to-day encounters with science and biomedicine that have shaped the historical and contemporary discourses, practices, and institutions of Chinese medicine. In our past conversations in Shanghai, she repeatedly voiced her concerns over the current debates about the relations between science, biomedicine, and traditional Chinese medicine among practitioners in Shanghai. Yet there we were, at a global conference in San Francisco, engaged in a conversation about the current state and future orientation of traditional Chinese medicine. There, national boundaries were sharpened and national consciousness heightened rather than dissolved (not everybody who was invited to the conference was able to cross the Pacific), and the questions of medical and cultural authenticity and authority were recast in national-cultural terms. Like many other practitioners from China, Xu was excited about the interests in Chinese medicine from those outside of China, and she was thrilled by the possibilities of forging new and growing transnational alliances of traditional Chinese medicine. At the same time, she was also concerned about China's place in the emergent new world of traditional Chinese medicine. She struggled to find ways of presenting traditional Chinese medicine in China favorably in relation to traditional Chinese medicine in the United States.

It was out of this particular context of encounter that deliberately simplistic, binary presentations of "China" and "the United States," the "Chinese" and the "Americans," "Chinese culture" and "American culture" were articulated and deployed. In other words, my conversation with Dr. Xu suggests that "China," "Chinese culture," and "traditional Chinese medicine" were not building blocks upon which a system of differences could be built; rather, they were relationally produced from particular sociohistorical locations and encounters.

While affirming China as the home to Chinese culture and firmly locating authentic traditional Chinese medicine within China, Xu saw no contradiction in stating that the future of traditional Chinese medicine was in the direction of "science"—bioscience, to be exact. For her, the bioscientific orientation, exemplified by courses in life sciences and molecular biology in particular, would not hurt the integrity of traditional Chinese medicine.

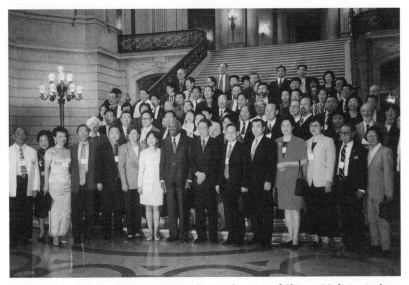

Participants at the U.S.-China Summit on the Development of Chinese Medicine in the Twenty-first Century, San Francisco, April 1, 2000. Photo by the author.

Instead, it would strengthen the position of traditional Chinese medicine in its competition with biomedical practices and institutions such as the two biomedical universities in Shanghai.

By insisting on and even naturalizing the nexus between China, Chinese culture, and traditional Chinese medicine, Xu was able to envision and pursue a future in bioscientific research without, in her view, compromising the authenticity of traditional Chinese medicine. While this strategy works for many practitioners arriving in the United States from China, it is far from unproblematic. In what follows I discuss the ways in which students of traditional Chinese medicine in the San Francisco Bay Area reinterpret the relations between China, Chinese culture, and traditional Chinese medicine—discourses where science becomes more political and problematic for the authenticity of traditional Chinese medicine.

Politicizing Science

The American College of Traditional Chinese Medicine (ACTCM) was founded in San Francisco in 1980. Its founding president was a former biomedical professional. Since 1987 it has provided graduate education and offered a master of science degree in traditional Chinese medicine. Over the years it has earned the reputation of being one of the most well respected institutions of traditional Chinese medicine both in California and in the United States more broadly. My informants in Shanghai who have had contact with the college through visits and international conferences almost invariably praise it for its astonishingly fast growth and for the determination of its administration to expand and improve its educational and clinical programs.

In 1999 the college set up a clinic at the former campus of the Meiji Institution of Traditional Chinese Medicine, which had moved across the Bay to Oakland.[7] The college's main campus and community clinic, however, are located in the Potrero Hills of San Francisco—some of the steepest hills in the city. I found it quite an exercise to walk from the CalTrain station at 22nd Street to the college, although it was by no means an unpleasant walk. On a clear day, once I climbed to the top of the hills I would be rewarded with the stunning view of downtown San Francisco to the north.

The college is hidden among residential buildings. On my first visit I was able to distinguish it only by the American flag flying from a pole on top of the building. In front of the entrance gate there is a small garden in which a number of common herbs have been planted, including, among others, *cheqianzi* (plantago), *maimendong* (ophiopogon), and *shenma* (cimicifuga). The herbs are labeled in Chinese and in Latin. Inside the gate is the reception area. When I first visited the college there were pictures of past graduating classes on the walls, but during a later refurbishment the pictures were removed. The current space is more simple and spare with its furnishings of a few couches and chairs, along with a display of brochures with information about the college.

Outside of the back door and up a stairwell is the parking lot adjacent to the college's community clinic. Behind the glass door of the clinic is a scroll of calligraphy dedicated by the graduating class of 1987. It reads *renxin renshu* (kind heart, kind skills). The interior always smells like herbs, although occasionally when the door of one of the inside treatment rooms opens a whiff of moxa overwhelms everything else. Immediately to the left of the entrance is the faculty study room, which is shared by adjunct faculty. Most of the faculty have their own practices elsewhere, and over the years, the college has made a point of hiring faculty members trained in China as well as those trained in the United States.

There is a reception area with clinical record storage to the left of the entrance and a pharmacy to the right. I liked watching the students behind the counter of the pharmacy putting together herbal packages. Rather than the frenzied yet astonishing deft movements I would expect to see at a pharmacy in Shanghai, these students moved in elegant motions and, most of the time, at a leisurely pace. The clinic receives on average one thousand patients a month, and each practitioner sees about eight patients per day.

In the pharmacy the herbs are stored in wooden chests of drawers located against the wall behind the counter where the students work. Like many herbal pharmacies in Shanghai, the drawers are color coded according to their therapeutic properties. With great precision the students weigh out the herbs using a *chen*—a Chinese-style balance that requires great skill and patience. Although there is an electronic scale at the corner of the counter, it is rarely used. After weighing the herbs the student distributes them evenly into several file folders, where the number of folders depends on the specification of the prescription. Other herbs will be mixed in using the same procedures. Small bursts of excitement break out when unusual herbs are used—for example cicada skin (which bears striking resemblance to the insect itself) or beautifully wrapped bundles of tiny bamboo branches. Most of these herbs are imported from China and actually are of higher quality than those used there.

There are eleven treatment rooms, eight small and three large, in the treatment area behind the reception space. The small rooms contain one wooden treatment table, one small desk, and two chairs. The large rooms, called interview rooms, are similarly furnished and are used for open sessions during which up to four students and interns study with the practitioner. Compared to the acupuncture departments in Shanghai, the spatial arrangements in the clinic are more private. The dean of the clinic, Cheryl Sterling, asks students to speak softly for the sake of privacy and to minimize disturbances. I spent most of my time at the college in one of the larger treatment rooms with Cheryl and her students, all of whom generously shared their time and knowledge with me.

Most of the therapeutic processes take place in the treatment rooms, although after interviewing the patients the practitioner and the students retreat to the student study room in the back of the clinic to discuss the treatment plan, while the patient undresses and prepares for acupuncture. To the right of the door in the treatment room where I did most of my work was a desk holding acupuncture needles, the needle disposal container, a stick of moxa, therapeutic massage oil, alcohol wipes, glass cups (for cupping), and a radio (which was sometimes turned on, at the patience's request, during acupuncture). The right half of the room holds a wooden treatment table, covered with disposable paper. Next to the table is an infrared lamp and a fan—the lamp is used to keep the patient warm and the fan helps to disperse the smell of moxa when it is overpowering. On the left side of the room is an office desk. Interestingly, the patient is invited to sit behind the desk while Cheryl herself sits in front of it—a reversal of the usual positions of interviewer and interviewed. Chairs placed along the sides of the desk are for the students to use during the interviews. On the desk there are two small pillows for pulse taking, and on the wall behind the desk is a poster of a Chinese peasant painting titled *Golden Lotus*. On the wall above the treatment table there is a print of an ancient Chinese painting depicting a group of horseback riders traveling through the mountains.

As at Shuguang Hospital, students at ACTCM play an important role in everyday clinical practice. Most of the students live in San Francisco or in nearby cities, although some commute from as far as San Jose. At the time of my fieldwork, the student body was predominantly white. Some of the students spoke Chinese very well—basic and medical Chinese is a language requirement at the college. In spite of this I witnessed occasions where two different conversations could be going on in the pharmacy—one in Chinese between a Chinese practitioner and his or her students and one in English between a white practitioner and his or her followers. Neither party seemed to understand or feel disturbed by what the other party was discussing.

The college's diversity in terms of ethnic background and medical training is considered by the students as one of its special features. Clinical styles are as diverse among those trained in China, the United States, and Europe as they are within these groups. While some students—especially beginners—find this diversity confusing, others love it because they can choose what kind of style they want to pursue. As some of them put it, "We got into Chinese medicine because we love having 'choices'—something you don't get with Western medicine. And what could be better than having such a wide range of styles to choose from?"

Not only do the students benefit from faculty trained in diverse styles, but also they are encouraged to study abroad. The most popular destination is China. Students who have been to China often come back from their trip amazed at how much they learned, especially in herbal medicine. Many students are told by practitioners—especially practitioners trained in China—that "herbs go much deeper (than just acupuncture)" and represent the essence of traditional Chinese medicine.

Not everyone, however, is ready to embrace China as the original home and authentic source of traditional Chinese medicine. Today, students who choose traditional Chinese medicine as their profession are not necessarily drawn to "Chinese culture" or "China." Many of them had some intense personal experience with traditional Chinese medicine before they decided on traditional Chinese medicine as their calling. Over and again I heard stories of how, after biomedicine had failed, acupuncture or herbal medicine "miraculously" alleviated their illness or the illness of a loved one—so miraculous, in fact, that they were compelled to pursue traditional Chinese medicine as a career.

In terms of personal and academic interests, some of these students are interested in "Eastern philosophy," some are drawn to alternative medicines, and others come from biomedical backgrounds but are interested in integrating acupuncture into their medical practices. In terms of their undergraduate training, some have degrees in the natural sciences while others majored in arts and humanities. Some students in the latter group complain that they thought they would not have to take science courses anymore if they pursued a graduate program in traditional Chinese medicine, but then were surprised to find out that courses in chemistry, biology, physiology, and anatomy were prerequisites for the degree program. Those interested in science believe that doing science entails having an open mind and therefore the willingness to explore new frontiers—which makes traditional Chinese medicine a rational career choice.

Even for those who are interested in "Chinese culture" (rather than, for example, alternative medicine as a whole), the linkage between "China," "Chinese culture," and "traditional Chinese medicine" is by no means taken for granted. One student who had just come back from China told me that her friends did not take the news of her China trip very well. As she recalls: "They were like, 'You are a Buddhist. How could you like China?!'" Among the Buddhist communities (especially those interested in Tibetan Buddhism) in the Bay Area the representations of the repression of various "spiritual movements" by the Chinese government have not worked in favor of China.

Furthermore, processes of scientization, which, as described above, Dr. Xu did not consider problematic in her commentary on the authenticity of traditional Chinese medicine in China, can pose vexed issues for students in California who try to understand what counts as "real" traditional Chinese medicine. Many of the practitioners and students who have been to China are surprised to see bioscientific concepts and biomedical technologies routinely integrated into the everyday practice of acupuncture and herbal medicine, even as these travelers acknowledge that they learned a lot about traditional Chinese medicine in China. Others are less sympathetic. As one of the students, whom I will call Noel, put it particularly bluntly: "There is no authentic Chinese medicine in China anymore. The communists have made it into a science. They got rid of all the spiritual and philosophical components, which are what really made traditional Chinese medicine so special. But they destroyed Chinese medicine in China. No, I would rather learn from old Chinese healers here than going all the way to China."

Comments such as this one do not take for granted the nexus between China, Chinese culture, and traditional Chinese medicine. For sure, Noel's commentaries were shaped by popular discourses and practices of science, spirituality, tradition, communism, nation-state, and national culture. One cannot separate her words from the surging interest in spirituality among the young, liberal, mostly white, middle class in the San Francisco Bay Area. It is thus important to keep in mind that Noel's commentaries were articulated from a sociohistorical location different from the context—a celebratory international conference—in which Dr. Xu presented her understanding of the continuous linking of China, Chinese culture, and traditional Chinese medicine.

As I have suggested, for Dr. Xu the authenticity of traditional Chinese medicine was grounded in its roots in Chinese culture, which she located in China. In other words, Chinese culture—and hence China—authenticated traditional Chinese medicine. For Noel it was precisely Chinese culture—in particular its presumed ancient spirituality—that had come undone in China. Simply put, for Noel traditional Chinese medicine without spirituality was not really traditional Chinese medicine. I should also add here that whereas Dr. Xu's representation of Chinese culture consisted of, among other things, eating seasonal foods, Noel understood Chinese culture as a bygone romantic timespace marked by spirituality.

Finally, Noel invoked "science" as a politically bound concept and practice rather than a neutral system of knowledge. As Vincanne Adams (2001) noted in her work on Tibetan medicine, practitioners in Tibet often insist that what they do is science rather than religion; they thus use "science" to depoliticize Tibetan medicine. Yet this act of depoliticization, Adams's analysis suggests, is itself a political act aimed at gaining state tolerance and even endorsement. Noel's position on science vis-à-vis traditional Chinese medicine was a political commentary as well. What is different here it that rather than depoliticizing science she decidedly politicized it. A politicized science was then used to delegitimize traditional Chinese medicine in China.

While Noel and Dr. Xu differ drastically in their understandings and representations of the nexus between China, Chinese culture, and Chinese medicine, they both assumed and projected—at particular moments and through situated commentaries—a more or less homogenous notion of China. For them, China either has Chinese culture—however differently it may be understood—or does not. In these terms, therefore, Noel rejected China once and for all.

Other practitioners of traditional Chinese medicine in the Bay Area may be similarly troubled by the questions of China and Chinese culture, but they have not easily given up on the project of finding authentic Chinese medicine in China. Jay Fitzgerald, the acupuncturist whose misadventure at the clinic in Shanghai I described in chapter 3, is determined to look for real authentic traditional Chinese medicine even if it means going to places no one has gone before. In the following section I will discuss his visions of China, Chinese culture, and traditional Chinese medicine.

Unfulfilled Yearnings

At a lunch meeting in Palo Alto I sat with Frieda Stein, Jay Fitzgerald, and Jay's teacher—an older Chinese acupuncturist with whom Jay apprenticed for many years and still works closely. The topic had turned to traditional Chinese medicine in China because both Jay and his teacher had just returned from trips there. Jay continued to complain about his experience with traditional Chinese medicine in China. During his trip he visited a number of coastal cities, where he made a point of visiting the local hospitals and clinics of traditional Chinese medicine. He was not, however, entirely pleased with what he saw: "In Guangzhou [a southern coastal city close to Hong Kong], they treat local symptoms rather than overall constitutions. If someone comes in with a bad shoulder joint they would just treat it locally, even though the person is obviously very spleen- and liver-deficient. They just do not get at the root of the problems, whereas I would most definitely want to tonify spleen and liver. And deficiency syndrome (*xuzheng*) is so common there. Of course, in China people do not eat well. I guess it has something to do with malnutrition."

At that point I could not help but point out that the patients I saw in Shanghai were quite different. In fact, obesity had become a significant problem among children. Summer camps were set up for obese children, and acupuncture was often used for childhood obesity rather than for deficiency syndromes caused by malnutrition. Jay replied that most of the deficiency cases he saw seemed to be children from rural villages.

Our conversations continued as Jay and his teacher talked about what they saw on their trips, and they voiced their concerns over what they took to be biomedicine's complete takeover in China. Still, Jay did not lose hope: "One of these days I will go back. I bet that I can find some little old lady in some rural village deep in China who does *real* Chinese medicine. I shall be content then." What Jay articulated through this image of the little old lady is a particular vision of China—the mysterious and distant ancient land that stood still in time. If he saw China and Chinese culture as heterogeneous, it was a structured heterogeneity organized by a particular cultural chronology: whereas the coastal areas may be contaminated by recent Western influences including Western medicine, some places "deep in China" must have preserved more pristine versions of Chinese culture and medicine.

As I discussed in previous chapters there is no question that there are important regional differences in the institutionalized practice of traditional Chinese medicine in China. In addition, a wide range of therapeutic practices was excluded from the institutional versions of traditional Chinese medicine. To complicate the matter even more, as Xu put it, "Everybody in China knows something about Chinese medicine." What Jay brought into focus through his remarks, then, is the nagging question of where traditional Chinese medicine ends, and which one of the versions counts as "real."

But the question itself already indexes an essentialist desire for the truly primordial and authentic—a desire with distinctive old-school orientalist overtones. For Jay, authentic traditional Chinese medicine must be located in some distant timespace in China, even though he may never find it. His view is by no means a new articulation of the relations between China, Chinese culture, and traditional Chinese medicine. Jay's translocal traveling and encounters were entangled in orientalist imaginaries and in turn reproduced them. Jay's proximity to China made "China" seem more elusive and distant than ever.

I have discussed three distinctive yet overlapping cases of translocal movements and encounters in which differently positioned practitioners and students of traditional Chinese medicine articulate their visions and understandings of the nexus between "China," "Chinese culture," and "traditional Chinese medicine." At the global conference of traditional Chinese medicine, contingent and even uncanny alliances are forged, and they are mediated by rather than in spite of the disparate interests of various conference participants. At a local college of Chinese Medicine in San Francisco, students continue to debate the authenticity of the kind of Chinese medicine they learn, and they do so by taking apart the fragile links between culture, medicine, science, and politics. Even for those who have traveled to China, their traveling experiences sometimes distance them from "Chinese culture" rather than bring them closer to it. China appears as an unreliable starting point for a journey through Chinese medicine. Science serves to both authorize and undermine Chinese medicine. The relationship between culture and traditional medicine seems at best tenuous. Rather than serving as stable points of reference, culture, science, and medicine are themselves produced, contested, and deployed through translocal encounters.

China or Chinese culture is not the underlying conceptual or structural foundation for the worlding of Chinese medicine. Nor does the "global" promise a worldwide community of traditional Chinese medicine that transcends differences and specificities. Various discourses of difference persist through the worlding of Chinese medicine, while their terms shift and new forms of specificity emerge. Emergent "global" connectivities, in this sense, provide new occasions for translocal encounters in which spatiotemporal distances and disparities are imagined and inhabited in everyday discourse and practice. Our world might seem smaller because of new information and transportation technologies, yet coevalness does not follow as a natural outcome. Indeed, the "Chinese century" is as imminent as it is distant.

In spring 2003, just before the Lunar New Year, I received an email message from a friend who had been a student at the Shanghai University of Traditional Chinese Medicine. Along with the usual New Year's pleasantries, he forwarded to me a parody piece titled "The Absolutely Authoritative World Map, Shanghai Edition" (Juedui quanwei shijie ditu shanghaiban). The phrase "Shanghai Edition" instantly reminded me of the term *haipai*, the "Shanghai style" of perpetual curiosity, studied embracement, and partial domestication of things perceived to be novel or different—sometimes in surprisingly creative ways.

In keeping with the irreverent haipai tradition, the map took the liberty of reinventing and renaming after a different country or region in the world each of the nineteen administrative districts of Shanghai. Whereas the downtown districts became Britain, Germany, the United States, Austria-Hungary, France, the former Soviet Union, the Middle East, Italy, and Turkey, the five suburbs were relabeled South Korea, India, Brazil, Argentina, and South Africa. Chongming District, which is an island off the shore of Shanghai, was dubbed "Central Africa." The anonymous author of the parody explained that "like many central African countries, Chongming District is rich in natural resource and cheap labor, its people are simple and innocent . . . and there are many nature reserves."

This type of caricature was applied to each district-country. The description of the downtown Huangpu District, or

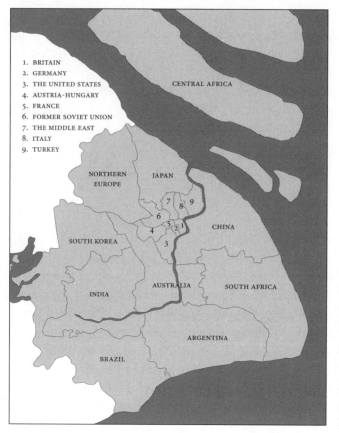

World map, Shanghai edition. Prepared by Tracy Ellen Smith based on "The Absolutely Authoritative World Map, Shanghai Edition."

Britain, reads: "Vintage [capitalist] country. Advanced economy. Prosperous commerce. It became even more powerful after annexing Northern Ireland (the former Nanshi District), and therefore a worthy representative of Shanghai. However, just like the Yellow River disappearing on the eastern horizon, Britain lost much of its luster, and has been surpassed by the United States." The United States, or Xuhui District, is located in the southwestern corner of Shanghai. Its description reads: "The hottest real estate market in Shanghai at the moment. Commerce is also very prosperous. Xuhui District prospered following Huangpu District, just as the United States took over from Britain."

Whereas the parody was quite astute in observing the shift in power relations across disparate scales—between Britain and the United States, and between Huangpu and Xuhui districts—it reserved the most vivid and optimistic description for Pudong District, the areas on the east bank of the Huangpu River where transnational finance and business quarters have been booming since Pudong's transformation from a largely rural area into a special economic development zone in 1992. On the "Shanghai Edition" of the world map, Pudong District became "China" and was thus described: "Without a doubt, Pudong best represents the development of contemporary China. Pudong fully deserves to be named 'China': rapid economic development, prosperous future, and full of energy and opportunities. However, Pudong lacks substance and does not have a lot of culture or romantic ambiance; all it has is one skyscraper after another. The native culture of Pudong has come into conflict with imported cultures, just like the native culture of China has come into conflict with imported cultures."

The "Shanghai Edition" of the world map was circulated among Shanghai's Internet communities as early as 2002, where it first appeared in real estate forums and later spread to a wide variety of sites including those for education, vacation, and football. The parody made no apology for its irreverence regarding geographic accuracy or for its crude and blatantly jumbled spatiotemporal narrative: indeed, it thrived on this irreverence. It managed to rearrange and deploy the world playfully and meaningfully and took great pleasure in doing just that.

This map challenges our habitual sense of scale and the order of things and places in the world (Ferguson 2006; Moore 2005; Raffles 2002; Tsing 2005). The author probably did not actually travel to all nineteen countries and regions identified on the map—and perhaps not even to all of the districts in Shanghai. Instead, the narrative draws heavily on reimagined memories of Shanghai's colonial and cosmopolitan histories, and it traverses, both decidedly and imaginatively, a wide range of spatiotemporal boundaries. It conjures traces of an older Shanghai edition of a world map—one carved up into foreign concessions. For Shanghai at the beginning of the new millennium, embracement and entanglement of the world still carry with them refigured memories of these more ambiguous and even painful varieties of cosmopolitan pasts.

Yet rather than reverse to an old world, former concessions have emerged in new forms in the "Shanghai Edition" world map. The world can be readily mapped onto the city of Shanghai, with both the United States and Britain reduced to its districts. At the same time, Pudong is not just a part of Shanghai or China but China itself—or, more precisely, China of the future. These are scale-making and time-warping tricks that subvert at once the order of the nation-states and normative discourses of globalization that posit the local and the global at two irreconcilable extremes of spatio-temporal scale.

The "Shanghai Edition" world map offers a seriously playful commentary on the shaping of the world that invites critical reflections. These mapping practices turn my attention to the projects through which entangled spatiotemporalities are made, rather than static maps of scale against which various translocal routes can be readily identified and measured. Its resolutely nontranscendental narrative of race, development, modernity, and capitalism highlights the gritty politics of difference that haunts emergent socialities of what makes up the world and at the same time recalls its shady pasts. It is a map in which the world comes to occupy the very heart of Shanghai, and is in turn "staged" (Karl 2002) in ways full of anxiety, irony, and hope.[1]

According to the map, the relocation of the Shanghai University of Traditional Chinese Medicine campus from Xuhui to Pudong District is also a move from the United States to China—and as such is in defiance of the out-of-China narrative that has so often been invoked to characterize the "globalization" of Chinese medicine. Rather than testifying to the triumph, novelty, or inevitability of global capitalism, the "Shanghai Edition" world map, as well as the shifting translocal trajectories of traditional Chinese medicine, reminds us of the workings of displacement, disjuncture, and meaningful contestation in translocal cultural formation. The worlding of traditional Chinese medicine entails dynamic workings of mapping, temporalizing, and positioning that cannot be simply described in terms of seamless and transcendental global circulation. It requires critical considerations of emergent world-making processes that depart from and go beyond narratives of global capitalism or liberal democracy.

This ethnography has not been about how traditional Chinese medicine transcends cultural and national boundaries and adapts to a new, globalized world. The authenticity of traditional Chinese medicine is not invariably tied to or locatable in remote times or distant places. Rather, these times and places are themselves fabricated and relocated through the worlding of Chinese medicine. These projects of time- and place-making are deeply enmeshed in shifting terms of difference that are both invoked and refigured in the always emergent worlds of Chinese medicine. At the heart of the encounters and entanglements of traditional Chinese medicine is a set of sociohistorically situated projects and processes by which people's visions, understandings, and practices of what constitutes the world—as well as how it is constituted—take embodied and protean shapes. Rather than contributing pieces of the puzzle to the uniform global map of traditional Chinese medicine, these translocal trajectories of Chinese medicine are always uneven. Instead of giving birth to one transnational or global community of traditional Chinese medicine, translocal encounters—whether real or imagined—provide occasions for constructing, negotiating, and contesting persisting cultural imaginaries and ways of making differences. In the end, the worlding of Chinese medicine adds up to both a little less and a lot more than a global map of traditional Chinese medicine.

Rethinking Science Studies

I entered graduate school at the height of the "science wars," when the relationships between social scientists who studied science and some of the scientists we studied were often tense and sometimes bordered on open conflict.[2] Those were difficult times, and yet they were also inspiring and galvanizing for a fledgling anthropologist like myself. I found myself able to ask questions about science that I had never been able to ask before, questions that were formerly unthinkable. Times have changed, however. Those engaged in science studies have learned to build constructive relations with those we study, and science studies—or rather Science and Technology Studies (STS)— has grown much stronger in terms of its institutional presence and scholarly impact. This shift does not have to dull the critical edge of cultural and social studies of science, or prevent us from generating new critical questions about knowledge production.

I still think that science studies is at its best when traversing seemingly discrepant sites in a manner irreverent to the boundaries previously drawn. I think, for example, of the work of the science studies scholars who venture into the sociological and anthropological studies of finance and those in the anthropology of finance who share similar analytical projects with science studies. As pointed out by Bill Maurer (2005a), emergent sociological and anthropological studies of finance that challenge the "inside" and "outside" of financial worlds and instead focus on form and performance bear striking analytical parallels to theories and methods developed in science studies (Maurer 2005b; Miyazaki 2003; Riles 2004). In fact, the sociologist Michel Callon (1998), who together with Bruno Latour was instrumental in developing the actor-network theory for studying science and scientists, pioneered innovative investigations into the finance world. The analytical parallels and overlaps between works about the anthropology of finance and science studies are indicative of another kind of boundary crossing. They are suggestive of the ways in which science studies can be rethought of as a form of inquiry—not a discipline bound to particular subjects of study, but critical and creative ways of posing questions and thinking through problems that travel across disciplinary boundaries.

My own intention in this book has been to bring science studies and medical anthropology into dialogue with each other without reproducing the hierarchy of knowledge that to some degree sustained the division of labor between them. Ostensibly, traditional Chinese medicine is not a "new" technoscientific object or practice in the sense that its professional identity has never been built on discovering or inventing the new. For Chinese medicine, novelty—whether technological innovation or new market environment and strategy—is always grappled with rather than embraced and advertised. But there is always something new about Chinese medicine in its everydayness if we look closely enough and if we are willing to broaden our sense of newness. The networks and assemblages of Chinese medicine have always taken me into both expected and unexpected directions by constantly probing and even subverting the boundaries between Chinese medicine and biomedicine, culture and science, old and new, local and global. My research and writing experience has taught me humility in front of knowledge: that it is much more than novel objects, textbook writings, or what happens inside the clinic and the classroom. My study of knowledge production has brought me face to face with effervescent discourses and practices of mapping, temporalizing, negotiation, and positioning that fill the interstices of everyday sociality. Knowing (in) the world is just part of being in the world.

Reimagining Anthropology

Much of anthropological inquiries and ethnographic endeavors today are set against the backdrop of globalization. "Culture," once a central subject of investigation and an analytical concept in anthropology, now seems an unfashionable conundrum that is all too often associated with hermeneutics and, worse, essentialism. The arrival of theories of globalization is both challenging and seductive for cultural anthropologists: that is, challenging in the sense that it shatters naive relativist notions of diversity, specificity, and difference that imbed culture within locality; and seductive in its promise to transcend the local and the specific, thereby making anthropology—which is assigned to dealing with the specific and particular within the global—relevant again in a new world of circulations and flows. But this salvation is at best only partial: difference remains entrenched in the local; it occupies an ontological priority within anthropology; and it continues to figure as the implicit starting point for ethnography and cultural analysis. Increasingly, then, there has been a suspicion that neither local nor global serves as a reliable point of reference for understanding human diversity and creativity in the contemporary world, and that metaphors of "circulation" and "flow" do not fully capture the uneven fields of power that both mediate and stall translocal connectivities.

It is with these issues and concerns in mind that I suggest an intervention by way of moving toward an ethnography of worlding. First, an ethnography of worlding does not privilege the ontology of dwelling over traveling. It is translocal in the sense that rather than taking "cultural difference" in its various ethnographic and theoretical incarnations as the starting point of anthropological inquiries, it emphasizes the ways in which various terms of differences are invented, negotiated, and deployed in everydayness. In other words, an ethnography of worlding conceptualizes difference as the contingent outcome rather than the starting point of translocal encounters and entanglements. Second, a focus on translocal encounters and entanglements helps us rethink globalization—or any totalizing narrative for that matter—as particular spatiotemporal arrangements that are always open to interested refigurations. These spatiotemporal arrangements involve processes of interaction, connection, displacement, and disjuncture, as much as they rely on circulation and flow.

Finally, if we can think of globalization as contingent and provincial spatiotemporal arrangements, we also open ourselves to the possibilities of imagining, understanding, and even making different worlds. Worlding is not a replacement for globalization. It is not a concept that aims to explain but rather is a way of asking different questions—including questions about things that have often seemed too "big" or out of reach for anthropology. Today the imminence of the "Chinese century" may appear more real than ever, just as the American empire once seemed the inevitable end of history. Many of us hold our breaths in anticipation and anxiety. It would be useful, however, to remind ourselves that the "global" is not always a very reliable map for locating the future, and that the problems with metaphors of the yellow peril, the communist takeover, or an emerging global economic giant are not that they are too wild but rather not imaginative enough.

NOTES

Preface

1. I use pseudonyms for practitioners and students of traditional Chinese medicine with the exception of public figures who are easily recognizable through well-known affiliations with particular institutions, through biographies and memoirs, or through public reputation for specific medical expertise. Most medical practitioners working at hospitals and clinics in urban China are graduates from universities and colleges of either biomedicine or traditional Chinese medicine. They hold at least a bachelor's degree in medicine, and some hold postgraduate degrees. After passing licensing examinations, both biomedical and traditional Chinese medical practitioners obtain the professional title of *yishi* ("doctor" or "physician") and are equally addressed as *yisheng* ("doctor") in everyday discourse. In contrast, the title of "physician" is defined much more narrowly in the American healthcare system, and "doctor" is most commonly reserved for those who have been trained at biomedical institutions and who hold the degree of Doctor of Medicine (M.D.). It is noteworthy, however, that in 1997 California Senate Bill 212 included "acupuncturist" within the definition of "physician." During my fieldwork in the San Francisco Bay Area, I noticed that patients sometimes addressed practitioners of traditional Chinese medicine by the title of "doctor," even though only a minority of these practitioners were M.D.s who, in their legal status as general practitioners, were allowed to practice acupuncture after additional training. Moreover, those yisheng who had immigrated from China often insisted that colleagues, students, and patients address them by the title of "doctor." My ethnographic account in this book follows the colloquial use of "doctor/Dr./ yisheng" based on my everyday fieldwork observation and conversation, and I mark an M.D. explicitly as such.

2. The Meridian Institute was in operation only a few years. According to Bob Flaws, a licensed acupuncturist, publisher, and activist of traditional Chinese medicine, the institute was promised a $2 million endowment from a single business man: "When his business went bankrupt, so did the Meridian Institute" (Flaws 2007).

Introduction

1. I use the terms "traditional Chinese medicine" (*chuantong zhongyi*) or "Chinese medicine" (*zhongyi*) throughout the book. I avoid the use of TCM, the acronym for the standardized and institutionalized version of traditional Chinese medicine, in order to keep in focus the heterogeneity and fluidity of traditional Chinese medicine and to highlight the fact that traditional Chinese medicine takes place both inside and outside of predictable institutional and pedagogical sites.

2. Peking Union Medical College Hospital was affiliated with Peking Union Medical College, founded more than a decade earlier. The hospital underwent a number of name changes to reflect shifting political atmospheres. Its original name was restored in 1985.

3. For reports from the initial trips, see "Herbal Pharmacology in the People's Republic of China" (American Herbal Pharmacology Delegation 1975) and "Acupuncture Anesthesia in the People's Republic of China" (American Anesthesia Study Group 1976). Both teams consisted of biomedical professionals and research scientists, and the reports were submitted to the Committee on Scholarly Communication with the People's Republic of China of the National Academy of Sciences.

4. The official definition of complementary and alternative medicine (CAM) by the National Institutes of Health is as follows: "CAM is a group of diverse medical and healthcare systems, practices, and products that are not presently considered to be part of conventional medicine. Conventional medicine is medicine as practiced by holders of M.D. (medical doctor) or D.O. (doctor of osteopathy) degrees and by their allied health professionals, such as physical therapists, psychologists, and registered nurses." The list of CAM practices keeps evolving; at present it includes such diverse elements as acupuncture, ayurveda, homeopathic treatment, folk medicine, natural products, megavitamin therapy, chiropractic therapy, meditation, and prayers for specific health conditions (Barnes et al. 2004). Acupuncture (though not Chinese herbal medicine) has been a perennial staple on this list.

5. The term *shuguang* means "twilight." Shuguang Hospital was established as Shanghai No. 11 Hospital in 1954 and renamed in the same year. The other two teaching hospitals of the Shanghai University of Traditional Chinese Medicine are Longhua Hospital and Yueyang Hospital. Putuo District Hospital has been recently added as the fourth teaching hospital of SUTCM.

6. One of these modern things is the stunning restaurant and recreational complex named Xintiandi. This project began in 1999 and was unveiled to the public in 2002. Featuring renovated early-twentieth-century-style *shikumen* architecture, Xintiandi has become a Shanghai landmark and a tourist destination. Interestingly, the Xintiandi complex also envelops the shikumen house where the first meeting of the Chinese Communist Party was held in 1921, a site that is usually ignored by tourists and those visiting the area's restaurants and pubs.

7. The Department of General Internal Medicine trains its own share of overseas students, although it does so at a slower turnover rate and in much smaller numbers compared to the Department of Acupuncture. These overseas students take part in

the regular four-year training program in Chinese medicine at SUTCM and are assigned to Shuguang Hospital for internships. Coming mostly from Taiwan, Korea, and other East and Southeast Asian areas and countries, these students are fluent in Mandarin. See chapter 4 for further discussion of overseas students at Shuguang Hospital.

8. Here I hold off from engaging in an account of "the social." I refrain from doing so not because I consider it irrelevant to knowledge production but rather because, as Latour (2005) has argued, our understanding of the social has become too predictable by assuming that we already know where the boundary between society and knowledge lies.

9. In Shanghai, the setup was ideal for conducting participant observation and informal interviews both during and between patient visits. My "internship" worked out well: practitioners were used to the presence of students and interns copying prescriptions, practicing acupuncture, and participating in the diagnostic process. Indeed, they were especially appreciative of my inquiries and attention, which they expected though did not always receive from their own students. In San Francisco, the classroom and clinic procedures were more formalized and structured. Compared to Shuguang Hospital, it was rare to have long lapses between patient visits: whereas patients at Shuguang Hospital simply walked in for visits that ranged from ten minutes to half an hour, the diagnosis and treatment sessions at ACTCM were usually prescheduled for a full hour. The students and faculty chitchatted only very rarely during the workday, and my interviews with them took place mostly during lunch or over coffee.

10. For example, some of the faculty members who teach at SUTCM also practice at a teaching hospital as well as in private or state-owned "expert clinics," and they regularly go to various neighborhoods to give free diagnosis and treatment. Many of the established practitioners in both Shanghai and the Bay Area travel across the Pacific on both official business and private tours.

11. The fact that my fieldwork was carried out in Shanghai and in the San Francisco Bay Area might lend itself to a literal reading of "multi-sited ethnography." Admittedly, the busy traffic of people, ideas, and things between Shanghai and the San Francisco Bay Area initially was an important reason why I chose these locales as my field sites: Shanghai and San Francisco have been sister cities since 1979; delegates from professional organizations of traditional Chinese medicine frequently visit each other in intellectual and academic exchange; and there is even an alumni association of SUTCM in the Bay Area. However, a multi-sited ethnography is not just about the enumeration of multiple places. To paraphrase George Marcus (2006), I think of multi-sitedness as an approach to places and subjects not as essential units of difference but as differently constituted, displaced, and hybridized.

12. Or, as Liisa Malkki (1997) calls it, "metaphysics of sedentarism."

13. In 1988 Gary Holmes and colleagues proposed a working definition of chronic fatigue syndrome (CFS). It was not until 1994, however, that the CDC agreed on and officially adopted the definition of CFS. Chronic fatigue syndrome has often been

associated with urban middle-class lifestyles, and at one point it was even nick-named "the yuppie flu" (Tuller 2007).

14. The arrest and trial of Miriam Lee was one of the turning points in the campaign to legalize acupuncture in California (see chapter 2 for further discussion).

15. On March 17, 1917, representatives of traditional medical communities from various provinces convened in Shanghai. Emerging out of this convention was the first national organization of traditional Chinese medicine, which coordinated efforts to promote guoyi and negotiate with the government (Qiu 1998). March 17 thus became "Chinese Medicine Day," which today is still celebrated by communities of traditional Chinese medicine in Shanghai and San Francisco.

16. Bridie Andrews (1996:202) counts seventeen schools of traditional Chinese medicine in Shanghai established sometime between 1905 and 1937 (although most were founded in the late 1920s). Some of these were minor academies that lasted just a few years. The senior physicians of traditional Chinese medicine in Shanghai today single out the prominence of *laosanxiao*.

17. In 1995 the Shanghai municipal government officially recognized fifty-six minglao zhongyi, all of whom were awarded a special stipend as well as an official plaque.

18. See Barnes (2003) for a nuanced analysis of a case in Massachusetts of the professionalization of acupuncture through politics within the community of traditional Chinese medicine as well as its relations with biomedicine.

19. To say that science studies have largely dealt with technoscience in Euro-American contexts does not mean that it has not been attentive to the politics of difference. To the contrary, there is a substantive body of work in science studies that addresses the racial, class and gender politics of scientific knowledge production. In addition, concerns with the practice, implications and consequences of science in developing and non-Western countries, especially issues of inequality and plurality, are familiar topics in feminist and anthropological studies of science.

20. See, for example, Kim Fortun's (2001) explication of global environmental advocacy after the disastrous chemical explosion in Bhopal, India, and Kaushik Sunder Rajan's (2006) query into the marriage of biotechnology and market mechanisms in India and Silicon Valley.

21. See Tim Choy's (forthcoming) examination of environmental politics in Hong Kong; Cori Hayden's work on bioprospecting in Mexico (2003); and Celia Lowe's investigation of biodiversity conservation in Indonesia (2006).

22. I here think of, for example, Vincanne Adams's (2001) examination of the complex relations between Tibetan medicine and discourses of science, religion, and the state; Jean Langford's (2002) query into fluid practices of ayurveda in postcolonial India; Lawrence Cohen's (1998) exploration of alternative knowledges surrounding Alzheimer's disease in India and questions of modernity; Stacy Leigh Pigg's (2001) work on the translational practices in HIV/AIDS education in Nepal; and many more. In the study of traditional Chinese medicine, for instance, Scheid (2002) invokes Pickering's idea of "bundles of practice" to think about the heterogeneity of traditional Chinese medicine and its problematic positioning vis-à-vis tradition and science, history and modernity.

23. *Zhongchengyao* or "Chinese formula medicine" refers to the factory-manufactured pharmaceutical products often based on commonly used herbal prescriptions. It usually takes the form of pills, capsules, or powder. In practice, Zhongchengyao products sometimes include biomedical components.

24. My friends at the university told me that the administration was adamant that the school should claim a spot in Medicine Valley. The ultimate goal of this move was to become a leading institution in both research in traditional Chinese medicine and, perhaps more important, the development of marketable products. As part of this effort the Murad Center for Modernized Chinese Medicine was founded. Ferid Murad, winner of the 1998 Nobel Prize in medicine, became interested in research on active ingredients in Chinese herbs that could be isolated and manufactured.

25. Most people in Shanghai and San Francisco, including practitioners of traditional Chinese medicine, biomedical professionals, and the general public, use the term "Western medicine" as the more popular vernacular for "biomedicine." This slippage itself is indicative of the conflation between the "Western" and the bioscientific.

26. In fall 2006, prompted by the news that South Korea was considering an application for World Heritage status for Korean medicine (which many Chinese believe to have come from traditional Chinese medicine), the Chinese government took a more proactive approach to its own application for World Heritage status for traditional Chinese medicine. Also see James Hevia (2001) for a nuanced discussion of China's push for World Heritage recognitions and the cultural and political complexity of this new cultural industry.

27. Anthropology itself has a tradition of offering divergent accounts of conceptions and practices of time and temporality (see James and Mills 2005); these include, for example, Clifford Geertz's (1973) account of spiral time in Indonesia or E. P. Thompson's (1967) thesis on the objectification of time during the Industrial Revolution. In philosophy there have been robust discussions of envisioning futures of radical ruptures and uncertainties—even as our pasts continue to haunt the present and beyond (Deleuze 1994; Grosz 1999, 2005). As argued by Elizabeth Grosz, time, although irreversible, can be understood as "an open-ended and fundamentally active force—a materializing if not material—force whose movements and operations have an inherent element of surprise, unpredictability, or newness" (1999:4). Both are powerful ways of rethinking time and temporality as contingent and formative. In the case of traditional Chinese medicine, however, neither approach seems adequate on their own in addressing the complex ways in which heterogeneous temporalities and worlds are produced and entangled. As suggested by Scheid, the past of traditional Chinese medicine, which takes shape in "entire libraries, living commentatorial traditions, and embodied lines of descent," enters its present as the past is constantly refigured through the future orientation of Chinese medicine (2002: 52–53).

28. In terms of ethnographic writing, Lisa Rofel (2007) has demonstrated how worlding highlights the complex ways in which the production of gendered subjectivities that place postsocialist China in a neoliberal world also hinges upon the imagining and reordering of this world.

1. Get on Track with the World

1. Housing was deregulated in China in the 1990s; formerly a social good allocated by work units, its deregulation meant that it became a commodity. Home buying, especially the purchase of the first home, was all the rage at the end of the 1990s in Shanghai. People sometimes jested that the question "Have you bought a home?" had replaced the more traditional greeting "Have you eaten?" The real estate sector continues today to be a mainstay in Shanghai's economy and social life. For young people and especially white-collar workers, however, car ownership, job security, and building substantive savings have joined home ownership as important factors in successful marriage proposals and negotiations.

2. These words have been noted by anthropologists and historians of traditional Chinese medicine (Scheid 2002; Taylor 2005), and they are widely quoted by governmental health institutions, practitioners, and even the general public in China. I was often struck by how easily they rolled off people's tongues—especially those middle aged and older. My most memorable encounter with this material was during a tour of the Museum of Traditional Chinese Medicine and Medical History at sutcm, where a copy of Mao's original speech was displayed in a prominent position toward the end of the chronologically organized display that began with the neolithic period.

3. In his analysis of discourses of "race" in Chinese history, Frank Dikötter (1992) argues that after 1949 discourses of race in China were replaced by those of class (192). Whereas I concur with Dikötter that discourses of race and class are conflated in socialist China, I suggest that one cannot be reduced to another—whether race to class or vice versa. Both are referential terms of difference rather than discrete, stable categories.

4. Hutchison (1975) further notes that the idea of a common China-Africa identity was met with skepticism in Africa, as the Chinese who worked in Africa did not really mingle with the locals.

5. See Barnes 1995 for a detailed and insightful account of the varied "Chinese healing practices" in the United States since the nineteenth century.

6. U.S. census figures from 2000 show that over the last decade California's non-Hispanic white population shrank to 46.7 percent while the percentage of Hispanic and Asian minorities grew at rapid rates. The size of the African American population changed little. California also had the highest proportion (4.7 percent) of people in any large state who indicated that they belong to more than one race.

7. The fall 2006 enrollment data from the U.S. Department of Education shows that at the American College of Traditional Chinese Medicine, 62 percent of the 255 enrolled students were "white, non-Hispanic," 2 percent were "black, non-Hispanic," 6 percent were "Hispanic," and 27 percent were "Asian/Pacific Islander." Those identified as "race/ethnicity unknown" and "non-resident alien" make up the other 2 percent (National Center for Education Statistics 2007).

8. There are many examples of these histories and biographies. For example, *Memoirs with Laurels* was a collective memoir authored by Dr. Bea Chi Pien, Dr. Kang Nan Yue, and Dr. Miriam Lee, and edited by the American Foundation of Traditional

Chinese Medicine and the California Chamber for the History of Chinese Medicine. The authors were prominent practitioners of traditional Chinese medicine who immigrated to California after the communist revolution in China. The book was published in Chinese by the Academy of Chinese Medicine, headed by Dr. DaRen Chen of Fremont, California. As a volunteer at the American Foundation of Traditional Chinese Medicine and in my capacity as a native Chinese speaker, I participated in the efforts to negotiate a collaboration. There are many other publications in Chinese—for example, a special publication by the California Certified Acupuncturists Association in commemoration of the twenty-second anniversary of the legalization of acupuncture in California. Chen Yong, a graduate of SUTCM who immigrated to San Francisco in the 1980s, and Gan Qixin, an alumnus of the Guangzhou University of Traditional Chinese Medicine, were among the key figures behind the publication. Choosing to publish in English, Miriam Lee's own memoir, *Insights of a Senior Acupuncturist*, was printed by the Blue Poppy Press of Boulder, Colorado—a key publisher of traditional Chinese medical texts in the United States. Peter Eckman's *In the Footsteps of the Yellow Emperor: Tracing the History of Traditional Acupuncture* also bears mentioning as one of the widely read and most influential texts. Published by China Books and Periodicals in 1996, it offers a different account of the history of Chinese medicine in the United States. Eckman, an M.D. and a Ph.D. in physiology, was among many American-born acupuncturists on the East Coast in the 1970s who went to Britain to train with Jack Worsley, a pioneer in Five Element Acupuncture. This took place amid the frenzy over acupuncture in the United States and when traveling to and extensive stay in China was highly restricted. Eckman has practiced acupuncture in the San Francisco Bay Area since the 1970s.

9. Major insurance companies and HMOs that cover acupuncture include BlueCross BlueShield, Kaiser Permanente, and Lifeguard, among others. The medical school at Stanford University as well as at the University of California at San Francisco both offer courses on acupuncture and other alternative therapies. The Bay Area hospitals that have acupuncture clinics or services include California Pacific Health Center, Chinese Hospital, and St. Luke's Hospital. At the same time, practitioners of traditional Chinese medicine, patient groups, biomedical professionals and politicians are working together to include acupuncture as a regular service at the San Francisco General Hospital.

10. To attract visitors to the booth, every once in a while Chu hollered out, "Want some information on Chinese medicine?" These moments made me feel more like a vendor than an ethnographer. See chapter 2 for further discussion of the commodification of traditional Chinese medicine.

11. Liisa Malkki (1999) also recounts the now-forgotten radical cosmopolitanisms that emerged after World War II. She notes the case of Garry Davis, a self-proclaimed nationless person who, rather than seeing the United Nations as the proper embodiment of a new world order founded on the sovereignty of the nation-state, insisted that the individual human being is sovereign and that all of humanity is the world government.

12. For example, Ken Wissoker brought to my attention the following anecdote and

new controversy surrounding the Maoist slogan "serve the people." In summer 2007, the American actress Cameron Diaz had to apologize for carrying a bag with the slogan "serve the people," written in Chinese, during a tour in Peru to promote the animated film *Shrek*. There, "serve the people" conjured bloody memories of Maoist insurgencies in the 1980s and early 1990s. One person's cosmopolitan dream is thus another's nightmare.

13. A few months later in March 2007, at the press conference of the Fifth Session of the Tenth National People's Congress (NPC), Li stated that on his recent trip to Africa, "seeing African people was just like seeing my own relatives." He also mentioned that since 1956 China had sent 160 thousand medical workers to Africa and treated 2.4 million clinical cases (Sina.com 2007).

2. Hands, Hearts, and Dreams

1. See chapter 1 for a description of how hospitals in Shanghai are divided into 3 divisions according to their scale, function, clinical and research strength, and equipment.

2. The term "herbal medicine" is thus a misnomer in that it does not reflect the wide range of materials used in traditional Chinese medicine.

3. Some prescriptions consist of only one herb. *Dushentang*, or "single ginseng soup," is a famous example. *Gaofang* (prescription of rich paste), discussed in the preface, is another example.

4. Herbs commonly used for the same syndromes (e.g., wind syndrome, dampness, etc.) are located close to each other. Ingredients used in combination in a ready-made prescription (*fangji*) also are grouped together. Ingredients often used in pairs in a prescription are stored in adjacent drawers or in adjacent compartments in a single drawer. For example, *jiegeng* (radix platycodi) and *zhike* (fructus aurantii) are often paired off in a prescription for the treatment of colds. Jiegeng has ascending properties (sometimes causing vomiting) and zhike has descending properties. They are always stored together in adjacent compartments.

5. Electric scales are used occasionally in herbal pharmacies in China, but more regularly at clinics of Chinese medicine in the United States.

6. In China and the United States herbal products are also available in powder and pill forms for easier and faster consumption.

7. See Farquhar 1994 for a thorough and insightful discussion of "syndrome differentiation and treatment" in traditional Chinese medicine.

8. There are four tones in Mandarin Chinese, each of which modifies a pronunciation to constitute a new meaning.

9. The "kidney" on the left wrist emphasizes reproductive functions, whereas the "kidney" on the right corresponds to urinary functions. See Kaptchuk (2000) for a detailed discussion of each "organ" of the zangfu system.

10. Yinyang is engendered by *dao*, or "the way." Yinyang relations also characterize the five-element system, a dialectic representation of all things in the cosmos. Certain schools of acupuncture and traditional Chinese medicine—notably the Worsley

school founded by the British acupuncturist Jack Worsley—take the five-element theory to be the most definitive feature of acupuncture.

11. See Scheid 2002 for a detailed discussion of the functional nature of the zangfu system.

12. Exceptions are made for those who are deemed "exceptional" talents (e.g., winners of major intellectual competitions or sports stars); these individuals are enlisted by prestigious universities without having to take the entrance exam.

13. For their part, the universities in Shanghai allocate a quota for admissions from other cities and provinces.

14. This system of hierarchy is a source of constant complaints from SUTCM faculty and administration.

15. See the introduction and chapter 4 for more discussion of the situational statuses of internal herbal medicine and acupuncture as contested "essence" of traditional Chinese medicine.

16. See Lee's preface in *Insights of a Senior Acupuncturist* (1992) for her own account of the arrest.

17. The Shanghai government banned zuotang in 2001 because of a public outcry against practitioners who used it as an occasion for promoting and selling expensive pharmaceutical products—the efficacy and safety of which were often problematic. It was not until 2008 that a number of reputable traditional Chinese herb stores were allowed to renew their zuotang practice.

18. Bridie Andrews (1996) notes that eye surgery and other minor surgeries were quite common in nineteenth-century China when Western surgery became a new sensation. The ascendance of surgery and waike in the late nineteenth century was not a matter of the diffusion of advanced technology from the West into China. Rather, waike became professionalized in China through a concurrence of and alliance with Chinese nationalist discourses, outbreaks of plagues, and individual interests in Western medicine and science.

19. Fuke is sometimes simply translated into gynecology. I avoid using this translation because the scope of fuke, which deals with a wide range of conditions related to menstruation, infertility, pregnancy, breast abnormalities, and so on, is much larger than the concerns of gynecology. Among all of the branches within traditional Chinese medicine, fuke arguably best exemplifies in a systematic manner that Chinese medicine does not target disease or rely on the identification of a particular disease as the prerequisite for medical intervention. It is not uncommon to see a girl or woman—more often in Shanghai than in the Bay Area—visit a fuke specialist to adjust her menstrual cycles, or treat conditions without the diagnosis of any "disease" or the expectation of being diagnosed with one.

3. Does It Take a Miracle?

1. Latour's two Great Divides refers to the divide between culture and nature, society and science, and the divide between the modern, western "Us" who supposedly maintain such a distinction and the premodern "Them/Others" who do not.

2. Whereas Latour inverts the roles of La Pérouse and the "primitives" at the end of his story, in the science fiction novel *The Calcutta Chromosome* (2001), Amitav Ghosh brilliantly subverts the story of the research for a cure for malaria by Nobel Prize–winning Victorian scientists. In the novel it was a low-class, low-caste female janitor at the lab who manipulated every step of the scientists' research in her own quest for reincarnation.

3. The surgeons and acupuncturists I talked to argued that acupuncture only produces partial anesthesia—a state in which muscles are not fully relaxed and therefore one that is not ideal for surgical operations. Although they concede that further experimentation may yield more effective ways of performing acupuncture anesthesia, they point out that new, steadily improving biomedical anesthesia drugs and procedures are readily available. Most of these drugs and procedures come from the United States.

4. According to historians of traditional Chinese medicine, the first of these yi'an appeared in the Han Dynasty historian Sima Qian's seminal work *Shiji* ("Historical Records"; ca. 90 BC), in which he recounts twenty-five clinical cases by a single healer (Fu et al. 1982).

5. For example, the curriculum at the Shanghai Professional School of Traditional Chinese Medicine included yi'an as a standard component (Qiu 1998).

6. In 1960 the No. 11 Hospital of Shanghai was restructured and renamed the Shuguang Hospital of SUTCM (Shi 1997).

4. Translating Knowledges

1. This treatment is called moxibustion. In fact, the Chinese word *zhenjiu*, which is often translated as "acupuncture," means "acupuncture and moxibustion." Moxibustion is sometimes performed without needling, in which case a lit moxa stick is held close to the skin without touching it.

2. In China, the seniority system at hospitals (including those of traditional Chinese medicine) follows the American model: doctors are divided into the categories of resident, attending, and chief in the order of ascending seniority and with corresponding duties.

3. See chapter 2 for a discussion of the resurgence of this idiom today.

4. Students in Shanghai sometimes complain that practitioners in their seventies and eighties often would not explain what they were doing, except to their own disciples. These complaints are justified to a certain extent. Older practitioners who worked in private clinics prior to the institutionalization of traditional Chinese medicine in the 1950s saw medicine as their livelihood and as something that needed to be protected from competition, even from their own students.

Even with the institutionalization of traditional Chinese medicine, many teachers continue to keep what they consider "secret prescriptions." With the marketization of the field in the 1980s and 1990s, an increasing number of practitioners begin to withhold what they consider their most personal and important clinical experiences and knowledge from students.

5. The fate of the shikumen forms a sharp contrast with old European-style mansions in the former concessions. Many of these mansions, especially those once owned by famous historical figures, have been revamped and turned into high-end restaurants, pubs, and cafés.

6. See chapter 5 for detailed discussions of the gender politics in and of traditional Chinese medicine.

7. See chapter 1 for discussions of how African students complained about experiences of racism during their stay in China.

8. Table 2 shows a clinic record for a returning patient, and therefore some of its categories are different from those on the clinic record of a first-time visitor. Note that acupuncture points are listed in both Chinese pinyin and English.

9. Huashan Hospital is one of the teaching hospitals of Shanghai Medical University.

5. Engendering Families and Knowledges

1. Wong and Wu's book, *History of Chinese Medicine: Being a Chronicle of Medical Happenings in China from Ancient Times to the Present Period*, was first published in Shanghai in 1932. The authors decided to compile the book because they were concerned about the lack of attention given to China in medical histories published in the West.

2. Legend has it that Shennong tasted a hundred kinds of plants to determine which ones were edible, which ones were therapeutic, and which ones could be domesticated—hence the popular Chinese saying that herbal medicine and food came from the same origin (*yaoshi tongyuan*).

3. See chapter 2 for a discussion of *waike*.

4. See also Scheid's account of families of practitioners from Menghe, a Jiangsu Province town just north of Shanghai, and the emergence of Menghe-style Chinese medicine (2007).

5. There were twenty-one women and eighty-five men in the 1956 incoming cohort, twenty-two women and eighty-one men in the 1957 cohort, and thirty women and eighty-two men in the 1958 cohort (Shi 1997).

6. Collier and Yanagisako (1987) argue that Bourdieu's model is useful for understanding how ordinary people realize the structure of inequality that constrain their possibilities. But Bourdieu fails to give an account of how people may also alter these structures.

7. Zhu Nansun was the granddaughter of Zhu Nanshan, a renowned healer (see chapter 3). Lin Yaoxing came from a family of fifteen generations of literati doctors. Chen Zhicai's father was a practitioner in the rural area surrounding the city of Shanghai.

8. The events that Pang refers to here took place in 1937 during the Japanese invasion of China. After Pearl Harbor and the beginning of the war in the Pacific, the Japanese also took over the European concessions in Shanghai.

9. The Union Medical College Hospital was set up by the Rockefeller Foundation, which was a crucial player in building the biomedical healthcare system in China (see the introduction).

10. Shimu, or "teacher mother," refers to the teacher's wife but never to a female teacher or mentor.

11. Note that I have disguised all of the names in this very famous family.

12. Dong Yixin had a third son, who never became nearly as accomplished as his elder brother or his nephew. One memoir says that this third son was the son of a concubine, and as such the son was too young at the time of Dong's death to be properly trained by his father. However, most biographies say that this third son was born to Dong's third wife, whom he married after the deaths of his first two wives, and that this third son was in fact three years older than Runhua.

13. See the introduction for an account of James Reston's encounter with acupuncture anesthesia.

14. This account is based on an interview with Barbara Bernie. On the West Coast the arrest of Miriam Lee and a few other Chinese American acupuncturists for practicing without a license had a similar effect.

15. Zhongxi Girls' School is the Chinese name of McTyeire School for Girls, which was founded by the Southern Methodist Mission and opened in 1892. The school was named after Bishop Holland McTyeire, one of the founders of Vanderbilt University.

16. Even though the story of Dong Yixin's daughter indexes the rift between different generations, genders, and medicines, it bears mentioning that it was her family who sent her to a missionary school in the first place. Furthermore, in telling me about her own life and career, Hsiang stressed that her father's family was "very open-minded."

6. Discrepant Distances

1. The Chinese, however, were quick to say that China does not have the kind of financial dominance to influence the global stock market (Sina.com 2007).

2. The CITIC building is named after the China International Trust and Investment Industrial Company; Printemps is an upscale department store headquartered in France; and Isetan is a Japanese-owned department store.

3. The economic crisis of 1997 and 1998 was set off, to a large extent, by the speculative activities of international hedge funds. George Soros, for example, gained much notoriety among the Chinese during this time. Sweeping the countries of East and Southeast Asia, the financial and economic turmoil was named the "Asian economic crisis."

4. See Barnes 1995 for a detailed account of the kinds of Chinese healing practices in the United States (especially the Boston area) ranging from standard traditional Chinese medicine to Five Element Acupuncture taught and disseminated by the Worsley school in Great Britain.

5. As I discussed in chapter 1, when talking about "Americans," people in Shanghai mostly refer to those who are of European descent. On formal and official occasions Chinese Americans are referred to as "Chinese descendants" (*huayi*) or "Chinese with U.S. citizenship" (*meiji huanren*), and in everyday discourse they are sometimes simply called "Chinese."

6. Many Chinese classify various foods by their properties. According to one classificatory system, foods are divided into groups labeled hot, warm, neutral, cool, and cold. During different seasons foods of particular properties are consumed (for example, food classified as hot strengthens the body during winter and food classified as cool is good for the body during summer). The classification and use of herbs used in traditional Chinese medicine follows the same principles.

7. The move by the Meiji Institute out of San Francisco left ACTCM as the only college of its kind in the city.

Epilogue

1. Karl 2002 offers an inspirational account of how, in the late Qing Dynasty, a growing sense of Chinese identification with the non–Euro-American world made the world visible as a structural unity. Karl argues that the "world"—or rather, the Chinese sense of globality—was not a passive, already constituted stage or space. Rather, the world is "staged" spatially and temporally and that the redefinition of China and the world are unfinished historical projects (10).

2. See the edited volume *Science Wars* (Ross 1996) for more details. The tension culminated in the physicist Alan Sokal's "mock article" in the cultural studies journal *Social Text* and his subsequent revelation that the article was meant to be a hoax exposing the fallacy of science studies and what he calls "postmodernism." See Fujimura 1998 for a discussion of the whole affair.

REFERENCES

Adams, Vincanne. 2001. "The Sacred in the Scientific: Ambiguous Practices of Science in Tibetan Medicine." *Cultural Anthropology* 16.4: 481–541.

Alden, Chris. 2007. *China in Africa*. London: Zed Books; Cape Town: David Philip.

Alden, Chris, Daniel Large, and Richardo Soares de Oliveira, eds. 2008. *China Returns to Africa: A Rising Power and A Continent Embrace*. New York: Columbia University Press.

American Anesthesia Study Group. 1976. "Acupuncture Anesthesia in the People's Republic of China: A Trip Report of the American Anesthesia Study Group." Submitted to the Committee on Scholarly Communication with the People's Republic of China. Washington: National Academy of Sciences.

American Herbal Pharmacology Delegation. 1975. "Herbal Pharmacology in the People's Republic of China: A Trip Report of the American Herbal Pharmacology Delegation." Submitted to the Committee on Scholarly Communication with the People's Republic of China. Washington: National Academy of Sciences.

Anagnost, Ann. 1997. *National Past-Times: Narrative, Representation, and Power in Modern China*. Durham, N.C.: Duke University Press.

Andrews, Bridie. 1996. "The Making of Modern Chinese Medicine, 1895–1937." Ph.D. thesis, University of Cambridge.

Appadurai, Arjun. 1991. "Global Ethnoscapes: Notes and Queries for a Transnational Anthropology." In *Recapturing Anthropology*. R. Fox, ed. Santa Fe, N.M.: School of American Research.

———, ed. 2001. *Globalization*. Durham, N.C.: Duke University Press.

Barnes, Linda. 1995. "Alternative Pursuits: A History of Chinese Healing Practices in the Context of American Religions and Medicines with an Ethnographic Focus on the City of Boston." Ph.D. dissertation, Harvard University.

———. 2003. "The Acupuncture Wars: The Professionalizing of American Acupuncture—A View from Massachusetts." *Medical Anthropology* 22.3: 261–301.

———. 2005. *Needles, Herbs, Gods, and Ghosts: China, Healing, and the West to 1848*. Cambridge: Harvard University Press.

Barnes, Patricia M., Eve Powell-Griner, Kim McFann, and Richard L. Nahin. 2004. "Complementary and Alternative Medicine Use among Adults: United States, 2002." *Advance Data from Vital and Health Statistics*, no. 343.

Baron, Richard. 1985. "An Introduction to Medical Phenomenology." *Annals of Internal Medicine* 103: 606–11.

Boellstorff, Tom. 2005. *The Gay Archipelago: Sexuality and Nation in Indonesia*. Princeton, N.J.: Princeton University Press.

Borger, C., et al. 2006. "Health Spending Projections through 2015: Changes on the Horizon." *Health Affairs Web Exclusive* 61: 22 (February).

Bourdieu, Pierre. 1977. *Outline of a Theory of Practice*. Richard Nice, trans. Cambridge: Cambridge University Press.

Bowen, John. 2004. "Does French Islam Have Borders? Dilemmas of Domestication in a Global Religious Field." *American Anthropologist* 106.1: 43–55.

Butler, Judith, Ernesto Laclau, and Slavoj Žižek. 2000. *Contingency, Hegemony, Universality: Contemporary Dialogues on the Left*. London: Verso.

Callon, Michel. 1998. "Introduction: The Embeddedness of Economic Markets in Economics." In *The Laws of the Markets*. Michel Callon, ed. Oxford: Blackwell.

Catlin, Aaron, Cathy A. Cowan, Stephen Heffler, Benjamin Washington, and the National Health Expenditure Accounts Team. 2006. "National Health Spending in 2005." *Health Affairs* 26.1: 142–53.

Chakrabarty, Dipesh. 2000. *Provincializing Europe: Postcolonial Thought and Historical Difference*. Princeton, N.J.: Princeton University Press.

Chavez, Leo. 2004. "A Glass Half Empty: Latina Reproduction and Public Discourse." *Human Organization* 63.2:173–88.

Cheah, Pheng. 2006. *Inhuman Conditions: On Cosmopolitanism and Human Rights*. Cambridge: Harvard University Press.

China Daily. 2004. "Subhealth Problem Poses Threat." October 8. http://www.chinadaily.com.cn.

Chinese Academy of Social Science. 2007. *Green Paper on Social Security (Shehui baozhang lüpishu)*. Beijing: Chinese Academy of Social Science.

Choy, Tim. Forthcoming. *Ecologies of Comparison*. Durham, N.C.: Duke University Press.

Chun, Allen. 1996. "Lineage-Village Complex in Southeastern China: A Long Footnote in the Anthropology of Kinship." *Current Anthropology* 37.3: 429–50.

Clifford, James. 1992. "Traveling Cultures." In *Cultural Studies*. Lawrence Grossberg, Cary Nelson, and Paula Treichler, eds. New York: Routledge.

Cochran, Sherman. 2006. *Chinese Medicine Men: Consumer Culture in China and Southeast Asia*. Cambridge: Harvard University Press.

Cohen, Lawrence. 1998. *No Aging in India: Alzheimer's, the Bad Family, and Other Modern Things*. Berkeley: University of California Press.

Collier, Jane, and Sylvia Yanagisako. 1987. "Introduction." In *Gender and Kinship: Essays Toward a Unified Analysis*. Jane Collier and Sylvia Yanagisako, eds. Stanford, Calif.: Stanford University Press.

Croizier, Ralph. *Traditional Medicine in Modern China: Science, Nationalism, and the Tensions of Cultural Change.* Cambridge: Harvard University Press.

Deng Tietao. 2006. "Correctly Recognize Chinese Medicine" (Zhengque renshi zhongyi). State Administration of Traditional Chinese Medicine of the People's Republic of China. http://www.satcm.gov.cn.

Deleuze, Gilles. 1994. *Difference and Repetition.* Paul Patton, trans. New York: Columbia University Press.

Dharwadker, Vinay, ed. 2001. *Cosmopolitan Geographies: New Locations in Literature and Culture.* New York: Routledge.

Dikötter, Frank. 1992. *The Discourse of Race in Modern China.* London: Hurst.

Dirlik, Arif. 1994. *After the Revolution: Waking to Global Capitalism.* Hanover, N.H.: Wesleyan University Press.

Dower, Catherine. 2003. "Acupuncture in California." Center for the Health Professions, University of California, San Francisco.

Eadie, Gail A., and Denise M. Grizzell. 1979. "China's Foreign Aid, 1975–78." *China Quarterly* 77: 217–34.

Eckman, Peter. 1996. *In the Footsteps of the Yellow Emperor: Tracing the History of Traditional Acupuncture.* Beijing: China Books and Periodicals.

Eisenberg, David, R. Kessler, C. Foster, D. Norlock, F. Calkins, and T. Delbanco. 1993. "Unconventional Medicine in the United States." *New England Journal of Medicine* 328: 246–52.

Eisenberg, David, Roger Davis, Susan Ettner, Scott Appel, Sonja Wilkey, Maria Van Rompay, and Ronald Kessler. 1998. "Trends in Alternative Medicine Use in the United States, 1990–1997." *Journal of the American Medical Association* 280.18: 1569–75.

Elliot, Michael. 2007. "The Chinese Century." *Time,* January 22, 20.

Evans-Pritchard, E. E. 1976. *Witchcraft, Oracles, and Magic among the Azande.* Oxford: Clarendon Press.

Farquhar, Judith. 1987. "Problems of Knowledge in Contemporary Chinese Medical Discourse." *Social Science and Medicine* 24.12: 1013–21.

———. 1994. *Knowing Practice: The Clinical Encounter of Chinese Medicine.* Boulder, Colo.: Westview Press.

———. 1995. "Market Magic: Getting Rich and Getting Personal in Medicine after Mao." *American Ethnologist* 23.2: 239–57.

———. 2002. *Appetites: Food and Sex in Post-Socialist China.* Durham, N.C.: Duke University Press.

Farquhar, Judith, and Zhang Qicheng. 2005. "Biopolitical Beijing: Pleasure, Sovereignty, and Self-Cultivation in China's Capital." *Cultural Anthropology* 20.3: 303–27.

Ferguson, James. 2006. *Global Shadows: Africa in the Neoliberal World Order.* Durham, N.C.: Duke University Press.

Fishman, Ted. 2004. "The Chinese Century." *New York Times Magazine,* July 4: 24.

Flaws, Bob. 2007. "The Need for Endowments in AOM Education in North America." *Acupuncture Today* 8.7: 1, 35, 37.

Fortun, Kim. 2001. *Advocacy after Bhopal: Environmentalism, Disaster, New Global Orders.* Chicago: University of Chicago Press.

Franklin, Sarah. 1995. "Science as Culture, Cultures of Science." *Annual Review of Anthropology* 24: 163–84.

Freedman, Maurice, ed. 1970. *Family and Kinship in Chinese Society.* Stanford, Calif.: Stanford University Press.

Fu Weikang, Zhang Weifeng, Wang Huifang, Jia Fuhua, Gao Yuqiu, and Wu Hongzhou, eds. 1982. *Yiyao Shihua* (History of medicine). Shanghai: Shanghai Kexuejishu Chubanshe.

Fujimura, Joan. 1998. "Authorizing Knowledge in Science and Anthropology." *American Anthropologist* 100.2: 347–60.

Furth, Charlotte, ed. 1975. *The Limits of Change: Essays on Conservative Alternatives in Republican China.* Cambridge: Harvard University Press.

———. 1999. *A Flourishing Yin: Gender in China's Medical History, 960–1665.* Berkeley: University of California Press.

Geertz, Clifford. 1973. *The Interpretation of Cultures.* New York: Basic Books.

Ghosh, Amitav. 2001. *The Calcutta Chromosome: A Novel of Fevers, Delirium and Discovery.* New York: Harper Perennial.

Gibson-Graham, J. K. 1996. *The End of Capitalism (As We Know It).* Cambridge, Mass.: Blackwell.

Gillman, Susan, Kirsten Silva Greusz, and Rob Wilson. 2004. "Worlding American Studies." *Comparative American Studies* 2.3: 259–70.

Gilroy, Paul. 2004. *Postcolonial Melancholia.* New York: Columbia University Press.

Good, Byron. 1994. *Medicine, Rationality, and Experience: An Anthropological Perspective.* Cambridge: Harvard University Press.

Greenhalgh, Susan. 2001. *Under the Medical Gaze.* Berkeley: University of California Press.

Grewal, Inderpal. 2005. *Transnational America.* Durham, N.C.: Duke University Press.

Grosz, Elizabeth. 1999. "Becoming . . . An Introduction." In *Becomings: Explorations in Time, Memory, and Futures.* Elizabeth Grosz, ed. Ithaca, N.Y.: Cornell University Press.

———. 2005. *Time Travels: Feminism, Nature, Power.* Durham, N.C.: Duke University Press.

Gupta, Akhil, and James Ferguson. 1992. "Beyond 'Culture': Space, Identity, and the Politics of Difference." *Cultural Anthropology* 7.1: 6–23.

———. 1997. "Culture, Power, Place: Ethnography at the End of an Era." In *Culture, Power, Place.* Akhil Gupta and James Ferguson, eds. Durham, N.C.: Duke University Press.

Handler, Richard, and Daniel Segal. 1990. *Jane Austen and the Fiction of Culture.* Tucson: University of Arizona Press.

Haraway, Donna. 1989. *Primate Visions: Gender, Race, and Nature in the World of Modern Science.* New York: Routledge.

_____. 1991. *Simians, Cyborgs, and Women: The Reinvention of Nature.* New York: Routledge.

Harding, Sandra. 1998. *Is Science Multicultural? Postcolonialisms, Feminisms, and Epistemologies.* Bloomington: Indiana University Press.

Harvey, David. 1989. *The Condition of Postmodernity: An Enquiry into the Origins of Cultural Change.* Oxford: Blackwell.

Hayden, Cori. 2003. *When Nature Goes Public: The Making and Unmaking of Bioprospecting in Mexico.* Princeton, N.J.: Princeton University Press.

He Shixi. 1997. *Jindai Yilin Yishi* (Anecdotes in recent medical history). Shanghai: Shanghai University of Traditional Chinese Medicine Press.

He Yumin. 1990. *Chayi, Kunhuo, Yu Xuanze: Zhongxi Yixue Bijiao Yanjiu* (Difference, perplexity, and choice: Comparative research of Chinese medicine and Western medicine). Shenyang, Liaoning Province: Shenyang Press.

Heidegger, Martin. 1996. *Being and Time: A Translation of Sien und Zeit.* Joan Stambaugh, trans. Albany: State University of New York Press.

Heim, Kristi. 2001. "Shanghai Gleams as China's Crown Jewel." *San Jose Mercury News,* October 18, 1.

Hertz, Ellen. 1997. *The Trading Crowd: An Ethnography of the Shanghai Stock Market.* Cambridge: Cambridge University Press.

Herzfeld, Michael. 2003. *The Body Impolitic: Artisans and Artifice in the Global Hierarchy of Value.* Chicago: University of Chicago Press.

Hevia, James L. 2001. "World Heritage, National Culture, and the Restoration of Chengde." *positions* 9.1: 219–43.

Ho, Engseng. 2004. "Empire through Diasporic Eyes: A View from the Other Boat." *Comparative Studies in Society and History* 46.2: 210–46.

———. 2006. *The Graves of Tarim: Genealogy and Mobility across the Indian Ocean.* Berkeley: University of California Press.

Holmes, Gary P. et al. 1988. "Chronic Fatigue Syndrome: A Working Case Definition." *Annals of Internal Medicine* 108: 387–89.

Hsu, Elisabeth. 1999. *The Transmission of Chinese Medicine.* Cambridge: Cambridge University Press.

———. 2002. "The Medicine from China Has Rapid Effects: Chinese Medicine Patients in Tanzania." *Anthropology and Medicine* 9.3: 291–313.

———. 2007. "Zanzibar and Its Chinese Communities." *Populations, Space and Place* (special issue), Frank N. Pieke and Janet Salaff, eds. *New Chinese Diasporas* 13.2: 113–24.

———. 2008. "Chinese Medicine as Business: Chinese Medicine in Tanzania." In *China Returns to Africa: A Rising Power and A Continent Embrace.* Chris Alden, Daniel Large, and Richardo Soares de Oliveira, eds. New York: Columbia University Press.

Hutchison, Alan. 1975. *China's African Revolution.* London: Hutchinson.

James, Wendy, and David Mills, eds. 2005. *The Qualities of Time: Anthropological Approaches.* Oxford: Berg.

Jameson, Fredric. 1998. "Preface." In *The Cultures of Globalization*. Fredric Jameson and Misao Miyoshi, eds. Durham, N.C.: Duke University Press.

Jordanova, Ludmilla. 1989. *Sexual Visions: Images of Gender in Science and Medicine between the Eighteenth and Twentieth Centuries*. Madison: University of Wisconsin Press.

Kahn, Joseph. 2004. "China Courts Africa, Angling for Strategic Gains." *New York Times,* November 3, 3.

Kaplan, Caren. 1994. *Questions of Travel: Postmodern Discourses of Displacement*. Durham, N.C.: Duke University Press.

Kaptchuk, Ted. 2000. *The Web That Has No Weaver: Understanding Chinese Medicine*. Chicago: Contemporary Books.

Karl, Rebecca. 2002. *Staging the World: Chinese Nationalism at the Turn of the Twentieth Century*. Durham, N.C.: Duke University Press.

Keller, Evelyn Fox. 1983. *A Feeling for the Organism: The Life and Work of Barbara McClintock*. New York: W. H. Freeman.

Kleinman, Arthur. 1995. *Writing at the Margin: Discourse between Anthropology and Medicine*. Berkeley: University of California Press.

Knorr Cetina, Karin, and Bruce Bruegger. 2000. "The Market as an Object of Attachment: Exploring Postsocial Relations in Financial Markets." *Canadian Journal of Sociology* 25: 141–68.

Kondo, Dorinne. 1997. *About Face: Performing Race in Fashion and Theater*. New York: Routledge.

Langford, Jean. 2002. *Fluent Bodies: Ayurvedic Remedies for Postcolonial Imbalance*. Durham, N.C.: Duke University Press.

Langwick, Stacey. 2010. *The Matter of Maladies: The Ontological Politics of Postcolonial Healing in Tanzania*. Bloomington: Indiana University Press.

Larkin, Bruce. 1971. *China and Africa, 1949–1970: The Foreign Policy of the People's Republic of China*. Berkeley: University of California Press.

Latour, Bruno. 1987. *Science in Action: How to Follow Scientists and Engineers through Society*. Cambridge: Harvard University Press.

———. 1993. *We Have Never Been Modern*. Catherine Porter, trans. Cambridge: Harvard University Press.

———. 1996. *Aramis, or, The Love of Technology*. Catherine Porter, trans. Cambridge: Harvard University Press.

———. 2004. *Politics of Nature: How to Bring the Sciences into Democracy*. Catherine Porter, trans. Cambridge: Harvard University Press.

———. 2005. *Reassembling the Social: An Introduction to Actor-Network Theory*. Oxford: Oxford University Press.

Latour, Bruno, and Stephen Woolgar. 1979. *Laboratory Life: The Social Construction of Scientific Facts*. Beverly Hills, Calif.: Sage.

Lee, Ching Kwan. Forthcoming. "Raw Encounters: Chinese Managers, African Workers and the Politics of Casualization in Africa's Chinese Enclaves." *China Quarterly.*

Lee, Miriam. 1992. *Insights of a Senior Acupuncturist*. Boulder, Colo.: Blue Poppy Press.

Lei, Sean Hsiang-Lin. 1999. "When Chinese Medicine Encountered the State: 1910–1949." Ph.D. dissertation, University of Chicago.

Leslie, Charles. 1977. "Pluralism and Integration in Indian and Chinese Medical Systems." In *Culture, Disease and Healing*. D. Landy, ed. New York: Macmillan.

Li Haoran. 2006. *Shanghairen de Shimin Jingshen* (The spirit of city dwellers of Shanghai). Beijing: Chinese Film Press.

Lionnet, Françoise, and Shu-mei Shih. 2005. Introduction. In *Minor Transnationalism*. Shu-mei Shih and Françoise Lionnet, eds. Durham, N.C.: Duke University Press.

Liu, Lydia. 1995. *Translingual Practice: Literature, National Culture, and Translated Modernity—China, 1900–1937*. Stanford: Stanford University Press.

Lock, Margaret. 1988. "Introduction." In *Biomedicine Examined*. Margaret Lock and Deborah R. Gordon, eds. Dordrecht: Kluwer Academic Publishers.

———. 1990. "Rationalization of Japanese Herbal Medication: The Hegemony of Orchestrated Pluralism." *Human Organization* 49.1: 41–47.

Lock, Margaret, and Nancy Scheper-Hughes. 1987. "The Mindful Body." *Medical Anthropology Quarterly* 1.1: 6–41.

Lowe, Celia. 2006. *Wild Profusion: Biodiversity Conservation in an Indonesian Archipelago*. Princeton, N.J.: Princeton University Press.

Luo Jing. 2006. "Qichengduo Shimin Yajiankang" (Over seventy percent of city dwellers are in subhealth). Shanghai Online. http://ala.online. sh.cn.

Magnier, Mark. 2007. "China's Medicine Wars: An Attack on the Traditional Healing Arts Has Inflamed Adherents and Sparked a Debate about Western Healthcare." *Los Angeles Times*, January 8, A1, 7.

Malinowski, Bronislaw. 1948 [1922]. *Magic, Science and Religion and Other Essays*. Westport, Conn.: Greenwood Press.

Malkki, Liisa. 1994. "Citizens of Humanity: Internationalism and the Imagined Community of Nations." *Diaspora* 3.1: 41–68.

———. 1997. *National Geographic: The Rooting of Peoples and the Territorialization of National Identity among Scholars and Refugees*. Durham, N.C.: Duke University Press.

Mao Zedong. 1999. *Mao Zedong Wenji* (Essays by Mao Zedong). Beijing: Renmin Chuban She.

Marcus, George. 1995. "Ethnography in/of the World System: The Emergence of Multi-Sited Ethnography." *Annual Review of Anthropology* 24: 95–117.

———. 2006. "Multi-Sited Fieldwork: Five or Six Things I Know about It." Paper presented at the quarterly meeting of the Center in Law, Society and Culture, University of California, Irvine.

Martin, Emily. 1992. *The Woman in the Body: A Cultural Analysis of Reproduction*. Boston: Beacon Press.

———. 1994a. *Flexible Bodies: Tracking Immunity in American Culture from the Days of Polio to the Age of AIDS*. Boston: Beacon Press.

———. 1994b. "Anthropology and the Cultural Study of Science: From Citadels to String Figures." *Anthropological Locations: Boundaries and Grounds of a Field*

Science. Akhil Gupta and James Ferguson, eds. Berkeley: University of California Press.

Marx, Karl. 1972 [1852]. *The Eighteenth Brumaire of Louis Bonaparte.* New York: International Press.

Maurer, Bill. 2000. "A Fish Story." *American Ethnologist* 27. 3: 670–701.

_____. 2005a. "Finance." In *A Handbook of Economic Anthropology.* James Carrier, ed. Cheltenham, U.K.: Edward Elgar Publishing.

——. 2005b. *Mutual Life, Limited: Islamic Banking, Alternative Currencies, Lateral Reason.* Princeton, N.J.: Princeton University Press.

Ministry of Health, People's Republic of China. 2006. Press Conference, October 10. http://www.moh.gov.cn.

Miyazaki, Hiro. 2003. "The Temporalities of the Market." *American Anthropologist* 105: 255–65.

Moore, Donald. 2005. *Suffering for Territory: Race, Place, and Power in Zimbabwe.* Durham, N.C.: Duke University Press.

Moore, Donald, Anand Pandian, and Jake Kosek, eds. 2003. Introduction. In *Race, Nature, and the Politics of Difference.* Durham, N.C.: Duke University Press.

Nader, Laura. 1972. "Up the Anthropologist: Perspectives Gained from Studying Up." In *Reinventing Anthropology.* Dell Hymes, ed. New York: Pantheon Books.

——, ed. 1996. *Naked Science: Anthropological Inquiry into Boundaries, Power, and Knowledge.* New York: Routledge.

National Center for Education Statistics. 2007. *College Navigator.* http://nces.ed.gov/collegenavigator.

National Institutes of Health. 1997. *Consensus Development Statement: Acupuncture.* Washington: Government Printing Office.

Ni, Hanyu, Catherine Simile, and Ann M. Hardy. 2002. "Utilization of Complementary and Alternative Medicine by United States Adults: Results from the 1999 National Health Interview Survey." *Medical Care* 40.4: 353–58.

Ong, Aihwa, and Donald Nonini. 1997. *Ungrounded Empire: The Cultural Politics of Modern Chinese Transnationalism.* New York: Routledge.

People's Daily. 1954. "Guanche Duidai Zhongyi De Zhengque Zhengce" (Carry out the correct policy on Chinese medicine). October 20, 1.

——. 1963. "Mao Zhuxi Jiejian Feizhou Pengyou Fabiao Zhichi Meiguo Heiren Douzheng De Shengming" (Chairman Mao receives African friends and declares support for the struggles of Black Americans). August 9, 1.

——. 1966. "Zhongguo Yiliaodui Zai Feizhou Zhijiao" (Chinese medicine team at the corner of Africa). January 25, 3.

——. 1967. "Mao Zhuxi Pailai De Yisheng: Women Xin De Guo!" (We trust the doctors sent by Chairman Mao). January 20, 5.

——. 1970. "Quanxin Quanyi Wei Maolitaniya Renmin Fuwu" (Serve the people of Mauritania). February 10, 5.

Pigg, Stacy Leigh. 2001. "Languages of Sex and AIDS in Nepal: Notes on the Social Production of Commensurability." *Cultural Anthropology* 16.4: 481–541.

Piot, Charles. 1999. *Remotely Global: Village Modernity in West Africa.* Chicago: University of Chicago Press.

Polgreen, Lydia, and Howard French. 2007. "China's Trade in Africa Carries a Price Tag." *New York Times,* August 21, A1.

Pollock, Sheldon, Homi Bhabha, Carol Breckenridge, and Dipesh Chakrabarty. 2002. "Cosmopolitanisms." In *Cosmopolitanism.* Carol Breckenridge, Sheldon Pollock, Homi Bhabha, and Dipesh Chakrabarty, eds. Durham, N.C.: Duke University Press.

Pomeranz, Kenneth. 2000. *The Great Divergence: Europe, China, and the Making of the Modern World Economy.* Princeton, N.J.: Princeton University Press.

Qiu Peiran, ed. 1998. *Mingyi Yaolan* (The cradle of famous doctors). Shanghai: Shanghai University of Traditional Chinese Medicine Press.

Qu Jiecheng. 2005. *When Chinese Medicine Meets Western Medicine: History and Ideas.* Beijing: Sanlian Shudian.

Rafael, Vicente. 1993. *Contracting Colonialism: Translation and Christian Conversion in Tagalog Society under Early Spanish Rule.* Durham, N.C.: Duke University Press.

Raffles, Hugh. 2002. *In Amazonia: A Natural History.* Princeton, N.J.: Princeton University Press.

———. 2010. *The Illustrated Insectopedia.* New York: Pantheon.

Rapp, Rayna. 2000. *Testing Women, Testing the Fetus: The Social Impact of Amniocentesis in America.* New York: Routledge.

Reston, James. 1971. "Now, about My Operation in Peking." *New York Times,* July 26, 1.

Riles, Annelise. 1998. "Infinity within the Brackets." *American Ethnologist* 25.3: 378–98.

———. 2004. "Real Time: Unwinding Technocratic and Anthropological Knowledge." *American Ethnologist* 31.3: 392–405.

Rofel, Lisa. 2001a. "Globalization with Chinese Characteristics." Presentation to the Department of Anthropology, Yale University, April 10.

———. 2001b. "Discrepant Modernities and Their Discontents." *positions* 9.3: 637–49.

———. 2007. *Desiring China: Experiments in Neoliberalism, Sexuality, and Public Culture.* Durham, N.C.: Duke University Press.

Rose, Hillary. 1994. *Love, Power, and Knowledge: Towards a Feminist Transformation of the Sciences.* Cambridge: Polity Press.

Ross, Andrew. 1996. *Science Wars.* Durham, N.C.: Duke University Press.

San Francisco Focus. 1997. "Alternative Medicine Goes Mainstream" (special issue). March.

Sassen, Saskia. 1991. *The Global City.* Princeton, N.J.: Princeton University Press.

———. 1998. *Globalization and Its Discontents.* New York: New Press.

———. 2000. "Spatialities and Temporalities of the Global: Elements for a Theorization." *Public Culture* 12.1: 215–32.

Sautman, Barry, and Yan Hairong. 2007. "Friends and Interests: China's Distinctive Links with Africa." *African Studies Review* 50.3: 75–114.

———. 2008. "The Forest for the Trees: Investments and the China-in-Africa Discourse." *Pacific Affairs* 81.1: 9–29.

Scheid, Volker. 2002. *Chinese Medicine in Contemporary China: Plurality and Synthesis.* Durham, N.C.: Duke University Press.

———. 2007. *Currents of Tradition in Chinese Medicine, 1626–2006.* Seattle: Eastland Press.

Schneider, L. 1982. "The Rockefeller Foundation, the China Foundation, and Development of Modern Science in China." *Social Science and Medicine* 16: 1212–21.

Segal, Daniel. 2004. "Worlding History." In *Looking Backward and Looking Forward: Perspectives on Social Science History.* Harvey J. Graff, Leslie Page Moch, and Philip McMichael, eds. Madison: University of Wisconsin Press.

Shanghai Kangfu Zazhi. 1989. *Dangdai Shanghai Mingzhongyi Liezhuan* (Biographies of contemporary famous [traditional] Chinese doctors in Shanghai). Shanghai: Shanghai Kangfu Zazhi Press.

Shanghai Medical Insurance Bureau. 1998. *Medical Insurance System Reform in Shanghai.* Shanghai.

Shanghai Municipal Health Bureau. 2007. *2006 Niandu shanghaishi sanji zonghexing yiyuan, quxianji zhongxing yiyuan, shequ fuwu zhongxing yiliao feiyong qingkuang* (Report on the situation of medical costs among division 3 comprehensive hospitals, central hospitals at district and county levels, and neighborhood health service centers in Shanghai, 2006). Document index number AB83120002007022.

Shen Ziyin. 1976. "Dui Zuguo Yixue 'Shen' Benzhi De Tantao" (An investigation of the essence of kidney in the motherland's medicine). *Chinese Journal of Internal Medicine* 1.2: 80–85.

Shengming Shibao. 2006. "Jindai Bainian Zhongyi Sanci Lunzheng" (Three debates over Chinese medicine in the last one hundred years). http://news.sina.com.cn.

Shi Ji, ed. 1997. *Shanghai Zhongyiyao Daxue Zhi* (The history of the Shanghai University of Traditional Chinese Medicine). Shanghai: Shanghai University of Traditional Chinese Medicine Press.

Sina.com. 2005. "Qicheng Yiwu Renyuan Ceng Shou Weixie" (Seventy percent of medical professionals have received threats). http://news.sina.com.cn.

———. 2006a. "Zhongyi Tuxian Feicun Zhenglun" (Sudden debate over the elimination or survival of Chinese medicine). http://news.sina.com.cn.

———. 2006b. "Serial Report on the Beijing Summit and Third Ministerial Conference of the Forum on China-Africa Cooperation." http://news.sina.com.cn.

———. 2007. "Jiandao Feizhou Guojia De Renmin Jiuxiang Jiandao Ziji De Qinren" (Seeing people from African countries is just like seeing my own relatives). http://news.sina.com.cn.

Snow, Philip. 1988. *The Star Raft: China's Encounter with Africa.* London: Weidenfeld and Nicolson.

Spivak, Gayatri Chakravorty. 1985. "Three Women's Texts and a Critique of Imperialism." *Critical Inquiry* 12.1: 243–61.

Starr, Paul. 1982. *The Social Transformation of American Medicine: The Rise of a Sovereign Profession and the Making of a Vast Industry.* New York: Viking.

Sunder Rajan, Kaushik. 2006. *Biocapital: The Constitution of Postgenomic Life.* Durham, N.C.: Duke University Press.

Tambiah, Stanley. 1990. *Magic, Science, Religion, and the Scope of Rationality.* Cambridge: Cambridge University Press.

Taylor, Kim. 2005. *Chinese Medicine in Early Communist China, 1945–63.* New York: Routledge.

Thompson, E. P. 1967. "Time, Discipline, and Industrial Capitalism." *Past and Present* 38: 56–97.

Tisdall, Simon. 2005. "Beijing's Race for Africa." *Guardian,* November 1.

Traweek, Sharon. 1988. *Beamtimes and Lifetimes: The World of High Energy Physicists.* Cambridge: Harvard University Press.

Tsing, Anna. 2000. "The Global Situation." *Cultural Anthropology* 15.3: 327–60.

———. 2005. *Friction.* Princeton, N.J.: Princeton University Press.

Tuller, David. 2007. "Chronic Fatigue No Longer Seen as 'Yuppie Flu.'" *New York Times,* July 17, F6.

Unschuld, Paul. 1985. *Medicine in China: A History of Ideas.* Berkeley: University of California Press.

U.S. Department of Health and Human Services and the Food and Drug Administration. 2007. *Guidance for Industry on Complementary and Alternative Medicine Products and Their Regulation by the Food and Drug Administration* (draft guidance).

Wallerstein, Immanuel. 1974. *The Modern World-System.* New York: Academic Press.

Walsh, Conal. 2006. "Is China the New Colonial Power in Africa?" *Observer,* October 29, 9.

Wang Junxiu. 2005. "Guowuyuan Yanjiujigou Chen Woguo Yigai Gongzuo Jiben Buchenggong" (Research institution of the state council declares that our country's healthcare reform is essentially unsuccessful). *China Youth Daily,* July 28, 1.

Wang, Shaoguang. 2004. "China's Health System: From Crisis to Opportunity." *Yale-China Health Journal* 3: 5–49.

Watson, Rubie, ed. 1991. *Marriage and Inequality in Chinese Society.* Berkeley: University of California Press.

Watts, Jonathan. 2004. "China's Rise in Wealth Brings Fall in Health: Economic Reforms Lead to Growth in Stress-Related Illnesses." *Guardian,* September 21, 16.

Wilson, Rob, and Christopher Leigh Connery, eds. 2007. *The Worlding Project: Doing Cultural Studies in the Era of Globalization.* Santa Cruz, Calif.: New Pacific Press; Berkeley, Calif.: North Atlantic Books.

Wolf, Eric. 1982. *Europe and the People without History.* Berkeley: University of California Press.

Wolf, Margery. 1972. *Women and the Family in Rural Taiwan.* Stanford: Stanford University Press.

Wong, Chimin, and Wu Lien-The. 1932. *History of Chinese Medicine: Being a Chronicle of Medical Happenings in China from Ancient Times to the Present Period.* 2nd ed. Tientsin: Tientsin Press.

Xilu.com. 2005. "Yige Mingyi De Si He Ta Chengshou De Tuoma" (A famous doctor's death and the condemnations he endured). http://bbs15.xilu.com.

Xinmin Evening News. 1997. "Baixing De Qiwang" (Common people's expectations). January 5.

Yanagisako, Sylvia. 2002. *Producing Culture and Capital: Family Firms in Italy.* Princeton, N.J.: Princeton University Press.

Yanagisako, Sylvia, and Carol Delaney. 1995. Introduction. In *Naturalizing Power: Essays in Feminist Cultural Analysis.* Sylvia Yanagisako and Carol Delaney, eds. New York: Routledge.

Young, Allan. 1982. "The Anthropologies of Illness and Sickness." *Annual Review of Anthropology* 11: 257–85.

Zhan, Mei. 2005. "Civet Cats, Fried Grasshoppers, and David Beckham's Pajamas: Unruly Bodies after SARS." *American Anthropologist* 107.1: 31–42.

Zhu Kezhen. 1954. "Wei Shenme Yao Yanjiu Woguo Gudai Kexue Shi" (Why we need to study our country's ancient history of science). *People's Daily*, August 27, 3.

INDEX

"Absolutely Authoritative World Map, Shanghai Edition, The" (Juedui quanwei shijie ditu shanghaiban), 195–97

ACTCM. *See* American College of Traditional Chinese Medicine

actor-network theory, 22, 99, 100–101, 182, 199

acupuncture: Africa and, 38; biomedicine and use of, 2–3, 20, 104; biomedicine compared to, 51, 104, 159–61; in California, 48–51, 209 n. 9; CFS and, 10; China and, 4–5, 10, 39, 121–25, 129, 163–64; cupping procedure in, 122, 138, 187; described, 123, 212 n. 1; Dong family story and, 169; Five Element Acupuncture, 210–11 n. 10; gender issues and, 123–24; "get on track with the world" and, 25; legalization of, 10, 206 n. 14; moxa and, 121, 212 n. 1; moxibustion and, 3, 138, 212 n. 1; SCTCM and, 39, 124, 129; Shuguang Hospital and, 4–5, 121–25; therapeutic effects of, 1; translocality and, 164; in United States, 50–51, 104–5, 183, 209 n. 10; women practitioners and, 123–24

acupuncture anesthesia, 2–3, 104–5, 124, 212 n. 3 (chap. 3)

Africa: acupuncture and, 38; China and relations with, 59–61, 208 n. 4; globalist

narratives and, 19, 25; healing practices in, 73; preventive medicine in, 19, 25, 34, 38–40, 59–61, 180, 208 n. 3, 208 n. 4, 210 n. 13; racialized identity and, 25, 39, 42, 129–30, 208 n. 4; reimagined, 42; students from, 3, 4, 42, 129; worlding in, 24–25, 34, 37–42, 59–61, 180, 210 n. 13

AFTCM (American Foundation of Traditional Chinese Medicine), xi, 7, 51, 167–68, 205 n. 9, 208–9 n. 8

ai herb burning (moxibustion), 3, 138, 212 n. 1

American College of Traditional Chinese Medicine (ACTCM): authentic traditional Chinese medicine and, 193; community clinic at, 186–88; conversational pedagogy in, xi; curriculum for, 188; gender issues and, 148; herbal medicine and, 186, 188–89; history of, 185–86, 208 n. 7; students in, 82, 181, 188

American Foundation of Traditional Chinese Medicine (AFTCM), xi, 7, 51, 167–68, 205 n. 9, 208–9 n. 8

Anagnost, Ann, 39

Andrews, Bridie, 11, 12, 123, 206 n. 16, 211 n. 18

anthropology: medical, 6, 15–19, 68, 200, 206 n. 19; multi-sited ethnographies and, 1–2, 8, 205 n. 11; reimagining, 200–201

Anti-Imperialist Hospital, 2, 204 n. 2
ask (wen) diagnostic technique, 75, 210
    n. 8
authentic traditional Chinese medicine,
    10–11, 106, 183, 184–85, 190–92, 193
authority, 93–94, 117

Bai, Dr., 138–40
Barnes, Linda, 11, 46
being-in-the-world, 24, 200
Bernie, Barbara, xi, 9–10, 92, 104
*Biographies of Contemporary Famous
    (Traditional) Chinese Doctors in Shang-
    hai (Shanghai dangdai mingzhongyi
    liezhuan)*, 150, 156, 157, 158
biomedicine: acupuncture anesthesia
    and, 2, 104–5, 124, 212 n. 3 (chap 3);
    acupuncture compared to, 159–61; acu-
    puncture use in, 2–3, 20, 104; CAM and,
    20, 64; "clinical miracles" production
    compared to, 14, 26, 82, 92–94, 112–14,
    159–60, 171–72, 189; commodification
    and, 64, 65, 66–68, 81–82, 88; define,
    204 n. 4; Dong family story and, 169;
    "the East" contrasted to "Western med-
    icine," 170, 172, 173, 214 n. 16; facial
    paralysis cases and, 131–32, 134–36, 137;
    family background and, 151; feminist
    analysis and, 156; gender issues and,
    148, 153, 154, 156, 169–71, 172; health-
    care costs and, 66–68, 139; herbal
    medicine compared to, 20, 51, 84, 85,
    104, 115; ideologies in, 12–14, 37, 93–94,
    153, 206 n. 15, 206 n. 16; knowledge
    production and, 151; Parkinson's cases
    and, 133–34, 135 (table), 139; rational-
    ization process and, 160; in SCTCM,
    105, 112; in Shanghai, 14, 52–53; teach-
    ing traditional Chinese medicine
    using language of, 26, 125–26, 131–32,
    134–36, 137–41; use of term "Western
    medicine," 207 n. 25; zangu systems
    and, 76–77, 210 n. 9, 210–11 n. 10
body-mind connection, 56–57

Bourdieu, Pierre, 154–55, 213 n. 6
breast cancer treatments, 84, 85
breast fibroids treatments, 84
breathing and meditation techniques in
    Chinese martial arts (qigong), 50–51,
    167–68
"bridge of friendship," and traditional
    Chinese medicine, 179, 181–82

California: acupuncture in, 48–51, 209
    n. 9; CAM popularity in, 80; com-
    modification in, 65, 80–82; conversa-
    tional pedagogy in, xi; corporatizing
    medicine in, 48–51, 209 n. 10; imagined,
    31–32, 35, 52; imagined China in, 3–4,
    177, 179, 191; international proletariat
    concept in, 41; legalization of acupunc-
    ture in, 10, 20, 45–47, 80–81, 208–9
    n. 8; Meridian Institute in, x–xi, 203
    n. 2; preventive medicine in, 14, 25, 34;
    qigong in, 50–51, 167–68; racialized
    identity in, 46, 47–48, 208 n. 6; style
    of living space in, 31–32, 35, 52; tradi-
    tional Chinese medicine in, 10, 20, 27,
    45–48, 80–81, 181, 208–9 n. 8, 209 n.
    9; tuina and, 41; worlding and, 51. *See
    also* San Francisco Bay Area; United
    States
CAM (complementary and alternative
    medicine), 3, 9, 20, 64, 80, 204 n. 4
cancer diseases, 54, 84, 85, 91, 92, 108–11
carpal tunnel syndrome, 49, 50, 72
CFS (chronic fatigue syndrome), 10, 205
    n. 13
Chakrabarty, Dipesh, 23, 152
chaofang (copy the prescription), 126–27,
    147, 212 n. 4
Cheah, Pheng, 35–36
Chen Maoren, 145, 146–47
China: acupuncture in, 4–5, 10, 39, 121–
    25, 129, 163–64; Africa's relations with,
    59–61, 208 n. 4; authentic traditional
    Chinese medicine in, 10–11, 106, 183,
    184–85, 191–92; contrast with United

States culture, 183–84; economic and political ascendancy of, 37, 175–76, 193, 197, 201, 214 n. 1; healthcare costs in, 67–69, 82–83, 84, 86–87, 139, 211 n. 17; healthcare reforms and privatization in, 44, 52–59, 66, 67, 82; history of medicine in, 145, 181, 213 n. 1; imaginaries of United States in, 27, 44, 178, 179, 214 n. 5; imagined, 176–77, 178, 192–93; racialized identity in, 39, 42; spatiotemporality and, 179, 198–99; translocality and, 178, 179, 198, 215 n. 1; waike in, 83, 121, 146, 211 n. 18; worlding of, 39–40, 193. *See also* Shanghai

Chinese Academy of Social Science, 67, 81

Chinese formula medicine (zhongcheng-yao), 18, 49, 113, 207 n. 23

Chinese medicine (zhongyi), 5. *See also* traditional Chinese medicine

Chinese Ministry of Health, 4, 18, 21, 35, 101

chronic fatigue syndrome (CFS), 10, 205 n. 13

"clinical miracles" production: actor-networks and, 22, 99, 100–101, 117, 182; authority and, 93–94, 117; biomedicine compared to, 14, 26, 51, 82, 92–94, 112–14, 159–60, 171–72, 189; cancer diseases and, 54, 84, 85, 91, 92, 108–11; clinical successes of, 107–10; knowledge production and, 93–94, 117; liver diseases and, 54, 91, 112; science versus Other knowledges and, 15, 17–18, 93–94, 95–101, 116, 117, 211 n. 1; shenbenzhi research and, 101–2; sociohistorical processes and, 105–6, 117; STS and, 14, 15, 25–26, 106, 115–17; television dramas and, 91–92; traditional Chinese medicine and, 26, 91–94, 101–6, 110; trajectories and meanings of, 93, 101, 106; translocality and, 14, 15, 92, 117; universality of science and, 100, 103; yi'an documentation and, 107, 212 n. 4, 212 n. 5; yide and, 111; yishu and, 111

clinical records of patients, 125, 126 (table), 134, 135 (table), 213 n. 8

clinic visitors: in China, 120, 124–25, 134, 138–40; tours for, 2–3, 9, 45, 104, 124–25, 204 n. 3

coimagination, 1–3, 6, 8–9, 204 n. 1

commodification: biomedicine and, 64, 65, 66–68, 81–82, 88; California and, 65, 80–82; CAM and, 64, 80; of carpal tunnel syndrome, 72; corporatizing medicine and, 48–51, 209 n. 10; curriculum for SUTCM and, 78; damai diagnostic technique and, 84; fuke and, 84–85, 211 n. 19; getihu and, 73, 88; healthcare costs and, 66–69, 82–83, 84, 86–87; healthcare in China and, 66–68, 82; herbal medicine prescriptions and, 69–70; international proletariat concept and, 73; Marianne's career choice story and, 83–84; medical anthropology and, 68; medicalization and, 71–73; mengxiang and, 72, 74–75, 86, 88; mingzhongyi and, 14, 82, 84, 85, 107, 206 n. 17, 212 n. 4, 212 n. 5; rationalization process and, 68–69, 74, 88; renxin renshu and, 25, 64–65, 74, 84, 85–86, 186; Shanghai and, 65–66, 82–86; stress-related health conditions and, 71–72; students' career choices and, 77–80; syndrome treatments and, 70–71; traditional Chinese medicine and, 64, 82–84, 88; translocality and, 88; waike in China and, 83, 211 n. 18; worlding and, 88; xin and, 74, 79, 88; yide and, 65–66, 84; yishu and, 65–66; yuanmeng and, 86; zhongyi waike and, 83–84; zuotang and, 82–83, 211 n. 17

commodities, deregulation of, 31–32, 208 n. 1

communism, 9, 10, 11, 190, 204 n. 6

complementary and alternative medicine (CAM), 3, 9, 20, 64, 80, 204 n. 4

conferences, in San Francisco Bay Area, 179–81

conventional medicine. *See* biomedicine

copy of the prescription (chaofang), 126–27, 147, 212 n. 4

corporatizing cosmopolitan medicine, 48–51, 209 n. 10

cosmopolitanism, 35–36, 42–44, 59, 209 n. 11

Cultural Revolution, 2, 36, 40, 41, 57, 128, 136, 204 n. 2

culture, concept of: globalist narratives and, 200–201; San Francisco Bay Area and, 179; translational practices and, 119, 142; worlding and China and, 193

Cynthia's real estate story, 31–32

Dai Chunfu, 87

damai (pulse taking) diagnostic technique, 75–76, 84, 210 n. 9

Department of Acupuncture, Shuguang Hospital, 4–5, 121–25

Department of Cosmetic Surgery, Shuguang Hospital, 121

Department of General Internal Medicine, Shuguang Hospital, 4, 121, 127, 204–5 n. 7

deqi (get qi), 132, 140

Dikötter, Frank, 39, 208 n. 3

dislocations, 26–27. *See also* gender issues; spatiotemporality; translocality

dispersal metaphor, 177–78

displacement, gender issues and, 149, 153, 159, 173

divide. *See* two Great Divides

Dong family story, 164–70, 214 n. 12

dream (mengxiang) and commodification, 72, 74–75, 86, 88

"East," contrasted to "Western medicine," 170, 172, 173, 214 n. 16

Eckman, Peter, 164, 209 n. 8

education. *See* higher education institutions

Eisenberg, David, 51, 80

entrepreneurial individual (getihu), and commodification, 73, 88

"essence" of traditional Chinese medicine, 5, 12–13, 163–64, 183, 189

Evans-Pritchard, E. E., 95, 97–98, 116

"external medicine of traditional Chinese medicine" (zhongyi waike), 83–84

facial paralysis cases, 131–32, 134–36, 137

family background: biomedicine and, 151; gender issues and, 27, 146–53, 158, 164–66, 213 n. 7; of men practitioners, 146–49, 172; of students, 147; of women practitioners, 9, 147–48, 153, 157, 158–59, 172, 213 n. 7

famous doctors of traditional Chinese medicine. *See* mingzhongyi

Farquhar, Judith, 11, 37, 73, 114, 127, 150

feminist studies, 6, 15, 16, 128, 153, 154–56, 178, 206 n. 19

fieldwork: field notes and, 125–27; in San Francisco Bay Area, 3–4, 7; in Shanghai, x, 4, 5, 7–8, 77, 119–20, 204 n. 5, 204 n. 6, 205 n. 9; translocality and, 7–9

Fitzgerald, Jay, 106, 191–92

Five Element Acupuncture, 210–11 n. 10

France, 40, 67, 163–64, 195, 196, 214 n. 2

fuke (women's illness), 84–85, 211 n. 19

"fulfill a dream" (yuanmeng), and commodification, 86

Furth, Charlotte, 124, 152, 154

gaofang (prescription of rich paste), ix–x, 210 n. 3

Geertz, Clifford, 207 n. 27

gender issues: ACTCM and, 148, 159; acupuncture and, 123–24; biomedicine and, 148, 153, 154, 156, 169–71, 172; continuity and, 149, 156; displacement and, 149, 153, 159, 173; Dong family story and, 164–66, 214 n. 12; "the East" versus "Western medicine" and, 170, 172, 173, 214 n. 16; family background

and, 27, 146–53, 158, 164–66, 213 n. 7;
feminist analysis and, 128, 155–56, 173,
213 n. 6; gender defined, 155; gender
roles and, 159, 171; herbal medicine and,
123, 124; institutionalization of traditional Chinese medicine and, 146, 148,
149, 165; kinship and, 149, 151–55, 173;
knowledge production and, 27, 149, 151,
173; Liu's chosen family and, 159–64;
men and, 146–49; men practitioners
and, 123, 124, 146–49, 151–52, 154; mingzhongyi and, 14, 150–51, 156; Pang's
story and, 157–59, 213 n. 8; patriarchy
and, 148, 149, 151–52, 154; San Francisco
Bay Area and, 159; SCTCM and, 124;
shifu and, 161–63, 164, 214 n. 10; shimu
and, 162–63, 214 n. 10; socialities and,
149, 153, 157, 172, 173; students and, 148,
213 n. 5; translocality and, 170, 172;
women practitioners and, 148–49, 153–
54, 155–56
getihu (individual entrepreneurial)
practitioners, 73, 88
"get on track with the world" (yu shijie
jiegui) concept, 25, 34, 43–44, 61, 105, 176
get qi (deqi), 132, 140
globalist narratives: Africa and, 19, 25;
concept of culture and, 200–201;
cosmopolitanism and, 35–36, 59, 209
n. 11; described, 18–19, 21–22; dispersal
metaphor and, 177–78; flow metaphor
and, 177, 201; nature/culture division
and, 17–18, 95–98, 98–99, 116, 117, 211
n. 1; reductive globalism and, 6; spatiotemporality and, 6, 22, 23, 34; Third
World countries and, 14, 19, 25; U.S.
mass media and, 32–33
Great Britain, 40, 67, 195, 196
Grewal, Inderpal, 178
guoyi (national medicine), 12–13

hand holding, in traditional Chinese
medicine, 84
He Liren, ix–xi

He Shixi, 107–8
healthcare costs: biomedicine and, 66–68,
139; in China, 68–69, 82–83, 84, 86–87,
139, 211 n. 17; commodification and,
66–69, 82–83, 84, 86–87; equity and,
67–68; fairness in, 67; in United States,
66–68
healthcare reforms, in China, 44, 52–59
health insurance, 44, 51, 58, 82
hearing (wen) diagnostic technique, 75,
210 n. 8
"heart" (xin): described, 74, 79, 88; renxin
renshu concept and, 25, 64–65, 74, 84,
85–86, 186
Heidegger, Martin, 22–23, 24
herbal medicine: ACTCM and, 186,
188–89; biomedicine compared to, 20,
51, 84, 85, 104, 115; for breast cancer, 84,
85; for breast fibroids, 84; as "essence"
of traditional Chinese medicine, 163,
189; gaofang and, ix–x, 210 n. 3; gender
issues and, 123, 124; men practitioners
and, 123, 124; origins of, 145, 213 n. 2;
pharmacists' experience in, 70; prescriptions for, 69–70, 210 nn. 2–6; in
Shuguang Hospital, 70; for stress-
related health conditions, ix; therapeutic
effects of, 1, 49, 215 n. 6; in United
States, 104–5, 186, 188–89; use of term,
210 n. 2
higher education institutions: curriculum
for, 4–5, 78, 124, 145, 204–5 n. 7, 212
n. 5; entrance examinations for,
78–79; Meiji Institution of Traditional
Chinese Medicine, 186, 215 n. 7;
Shanghai Medical University, 53, 77–78,
101–2, 213 n. 9; Shanghai No. 2 Medical
University, 77–78. See also American
College of Traditional Chinese
Medicine; Shanghai University of
Traditional Chinese Medicine
hospitals: Anti-Imperialist Hospital, 2,
204 n. 2; division of, 53, 68, 210 n. 1;
gender issues in, 148; Longhua

hospitals (*cont.*)

Hospital, x, 53, 68, 82, 204; Peking Union Medical College Hospital, 2, 160, 204 n. 2, 213 n. 9; Shanghai No. 11 Hospital, 14, 108, 204 n. 5, 212 n. 6; Shuguang Hospital, 4, 14, 53; teaching, 53, 68, 82, 204; Yueyang Hospital, 53, 68, 82, 204. *See also* Shuguang Hospital

Hsiang Tung, 167–71, 214 n. 16

Hsu, Elisabeth, 11, 37–38, 61, 73, 127, 151

Hu Erxiong, 83–84

Huang Jixian: biography of, 128–30; biomedical language in teaching, 26, 137–38, 138–41; facial paralysis cases and, 131–32, 135–36, 137; Parkinson's cases and, 133–34, 135 (table), 139; translation practices and, 26, 137–38, 141; treatment rooms headed by, 121–25

Hutchison, Alan, 37, 38, 39

identities, 9, 26, 155–56, 172. *See also* racialized identity

illness treatments: acupuncture compared to biomedicine, 159–61; cancer diseases and, 54, 84, 85, 91, 92, 108–11; "clinical miracles" production compared to biomedicine, 14, 26, 82, 92–94, 112–14, 159–60, 171–72, 189; herbal medicine compared to biomedicine, 20, 51, 84, 85; kidney research and, 101–2; liver diseases and, 54, 91, 112; Parkinson's cases and, 133–34, 135 (table), 139; shenbenzhi research and, 101–2. *See also* stress-related health conditions

institutions: in China, 12–14, 37, 52–53, 206 n. 15, 206 n. 16; institutionalization of traditional Chinese medicine, 146, 148, 149, 165, 212 n. 4; translational practices and, 119, 141. *See also specific hospitals and institutions of higher education*

insurance, health, 44, 51, 58, 82

International Acupuncture Training Center, 39, 128, 129, 138

international conferences, in San Francisco Bay Area, 179–81

international proletariat, concept of, 14, 25, 34, 37–42, 59, 73, 103, 209–10 n. 12

jingluo system, 77

Jinqiu California Garden, 31–32, 52

Jiren Clinic, 110–11

jiuyi (old medicine), 12–13

"Juedui quanwei shijie ditu shanghaiban" (The Absolutely Authoritative World Map, Shanghai Edition), 195–97

Kaptchuk, Ted, 11, 74

kidney research, 101–2

"kind heart and kind skills" (renxin renshu), 25, 64–65, 74, 84, 85–86, 186

kinship: gender issues and, 149, 151–55, 173; knowledge production and, 149, 152, 164, 173; mentor-disciple relationship and, 127, 153, 161–62; shifu and, 162–63, 164; socialities of, 149, 172, 173

knowledge production: being-in-the-world and, 24, 200; biomedicine and, 151; "clinical miracles" production and, 93–94, 117; displacement and, 2; gender issues and, 27, 149, 151, 173; kinship and, 149, 152, 164, 173; science and, 14, 15, 18, 25–26, 116–17; socialities and, 200; spatio-temporality and, 24, 35; translational practices and, 26, 141–42; translocality and, 6; worlding and, 25

laosanxiao ("the three old schools"), 13, 148, 157, 166, 206 n. 16

La Pérouse, Jean-François de, 99–100, 101, 212 n. 2 (chap. 3)

Latour, Bruno, 17–18, 22, 95, 98–100, 199, 205 n. 8, 211 n. 1, 212 n. 2 (chap. 3). *See also* two Great Divides

Lee, Miriam, 10, 11, 60, 81, 206 n. 14

legalization of traditional Chinese medicine, in California, 10, 20, 45–47, 80–81, 208–9 n. 8

politicizing science, in San Francisco Bay Area, 189, 190–91

power relations and translocality, 11, 24, 195, 196, 201

practitioners: "clinical miracles" production and, 91–92; education of, 203 n. 1; gender issues and, 148; middle-class zhishifenzi, 40; pohai zhisi of, 40; in Shuguang Hospital, 121, 157, 212 n. 2; titles of, 203 n. 1; translocal activities of, 8, 205 n. 10

prescription of rich paste (gaofang), ix–x, 210 n. 3

prescriptions for herbal medicine, 69–70, 210 nn. 2–6

preventive medicine: in Africa, 19, 25, 34, 38–40, 59–61, 180, 208 n. 3, 208 n. 4, 210 n. 13; in California, 14, 25, 34; Shanghai yajiankang, 35, 45, 53–58, 66, 93; stress-related health conditions and, 45, 49, 51, 56, 58; worlding and, 36–37, 208 n. 2

privatization of healthcare, in China, 44, 52–59, 66, 67, 82

proletariat, concept of, 14, 25, 34, 37–42, 59, 73, 103, 209–10 n. 12

pulse taking (damai) diagnostic technique, 75–76, 84, 210 n. 9

qi (vital force): deqi, 132, 140; described, 1, 57, 115, 132, 168

qigong (breathing and meditation techniques in Chinese martial arts), 50–51, 167–68

Qiu Peiran, 13, 27, 148, 162, 206 n. 15, 212 n. 5

racialized identity: Africa and, 25, 39, 42, 129–30, 208 n. 4; in California, 46, 47–48, 208 n. 6; in China, 39, 42; imagined whiteness and, 42; international students and, 42; worlding and, 39, 42, 46, 47–48, 59–61, 208 n. 3, 208 n. 4, 208 n. 6, 210 n. 13

rationalization process, 68–69, 74, 88, 160–61

reductive globalism, 6

renxin renshu (kind heart and kind skills), 25, 64–65, 74, 84, 85–86, 186

Reston, James, 2–3, 104, 168

Rockefeller Foundation, 3, 204 n. 2, 213 n. 9

Rofel, Lisa, 36, 207 n. 28

Ruan Wangchun, 166

San Francisco Bay Area: acupuncture practitioners in, 27, 148, 159; Chinese biomedical students in, 181; concept of culture in, 179; concept of science in, 179, 193; concept of traditional Chinese medicine in, 179; field sites in, 3–4, 7; gender issues in, 148, 159; imagined China in, 3–4, 177, 179, 191; insurance policies in, 51, 82; inter-national conferences in, 179–81; po-liticizing science in, 189, 190–91; translocality in, 27, 192–93. *See also* American College of Traditional Chinese Medicine; California; United States

Scheid, Volker, 11, 74, 127, 153, 207 n. 27, 208 n. 2

science and technology studies (STS): "clinical miracles" production and, 106, 115–17; concept of science, in San Francisco Bay Area, 179, 193; cultural and social studies and, 199; finance studies and, 199–200; knowledge production and, 14, 15, 18, 25–26, 116–17; medical anthropology and, 200; politicizing science and, 189, 190–91; science versus Other knowledges, 15, 17–18, 93–94, 95–101, 116, 117, 211 n. 1; "science wars" and, 199, 215 n. 2; scientists as masculinist Eurocentric subjects and, 100–101; traditional Chinese medicine and, 161; universality of science and, 13, 15, 37, 100, 103, 140–41

"skill of medical practice" (yishu), 65–66, 111

smelling (wen) diagnostic technique, 75

Snow, Philip, 38, 40

socialities: authority in, 93–94, 117; complex and emerging, xi–xii, 1, 6, 12, 72, 184–85, 205 n. 8; of displacement, xi; gender issues and, 149, 153, 157, 172, 173; of kinship, 149, 172, 173; knowledge production and, 200

"softness" of traditional Chinese medicine, 64, 88

spatiotemporality: actor-networks and, 22; China and, 179, 198–99; "cultural difference" and, 27, 35, 201; globalist narratives and, 6, 22, 23, 34; knowledge production and, 24, 35; reconfigurations in, 182, 201; traditional Chinese medicine and, 22, 207 n. 27; trajectories in, 182; translocality and, 22, 193, 207 n. 27; United States and, 179; worlding and, 176–77, 198–99

Spivak, Gayatri Chakravorty, 23

Stanford University, xi, 9, 167, 209 n. 9

State Administration of Traditional Chinese Medicine, 20, 21

stress-related health conditions: facial paralysis and, 131–32, 135–36, 137; herbal medicine and, ix; magnets and, 48; medicalization of, 71–72; preventive medicine and, 45, 49, 51, 56, 58

STS. See science and technology studies

students: in ACTCM, 82, 181, 188; from Africa, 3, 4, 42, 129; career choices at SUTCM, 77–80; family background of, 147; gender issues and, 148, 213 n. 5; racialized identity of, 42; Shi Huizong's story, 77–80; in Shuguang Hospital, 4, 14, 40, 53, 168, 204–5 n. 7

subhealth (yajiankang), 35, 45, 53–58, 66, 93

surgery (waike), 83, 121, 146, 211 n. 18

SUTCM. See Shanghai University of Traditional Chinese Medicine

syndrome differentiation and treatments, 70–71

Tanzania, 60, 73. See also Africa

Taylor, Kim, 11, 37, 208 n. 2

"teacher-mother" (shimu), and gender issues, 162–63, 214 n. 10

television dramas, and "clinical miracles" production, 91–92

therapeutic massage (tuina), 41, 124

Third World countries: globalist narratives and, 14, 19, 25; worlding and, 14, 19, 25, 34, 38–40, 59–61, 103, 210 n. 13. See also Africa

Thompson, E. P., 207 n. 27

"three old schools" (laosanxiao), 13, 148, 157, 166, 206 n. 16

Tibetan medicine, 190–91

tours for clinic visitors, 2–3, 9, 45, 104, 124–25, 204 n. 3

traditional Chinese medicine: as "bridge of friendship," 179, 181–82; change and, 10–11; debunking of, xi, 9; described, 1, 94; "essence" of, 5, 12–13, 163–64, 183, 189; everydayness of, 12; history of, 12–15, 181; innovation in, 200; reinvention of, in California, 20, 45–48, 208–9 n. 8; scientific basis for, 161; therapeutic effects of, 1; as treasure, 37, 181; unbinding of, 9–15; use of TCM, 204 n. 1; zhongyi and, 5

translational practices: biomedicine language in teaching traditional Chinese medicine, 26, 125–26, 131–32, 134–36, 137–41; clinical records of patients and, 125, 126 (table), 134, 135 (table), 213 n. 8; clinic visitors and, 124–25, 134, 138–40; cultural translations and, 119, 142; facial paralysis cases and, 131–32, 134–36, 137; field notes and, 125–27; institutional sites and, 119, 141; knowledge production and, 26, 141–42; meaning production and, 26, 141–42; Parkinson's cases and, 133–34, 135 (table), 139; sociohistorical identities and, 26; worlding "tradition" and, 130–31

translocality: acupuncture and, 164;

worling: Africa and, 24–25, 34, 37–42, 59–61, 180, 210 n. 13; authorities of traditional Chinese medicine and, 25, 193; California and, 51; commodification and, 88; described, 7, 19, 24; displacement and, 7; emergent, 22, 198; ethnography of, 22–24; knowledge production and, 25; preventive medicine and, 36–37, 208 n. 2; racialized identity and, 39, 42, 46, 47–48, 59–61, 208 n. 3, 208 n. 4, 208 n. 6, 210 n. 13; spatiotemporality and, 176–77, 198–99; SUTCM and, 39; Third World countries and, 14, 19, 25, 34, 38–40, 59–61, 103, 210 n. 13; of traditional Chinese medicine, 22, 130–31; trajectories and discontinuities in, 172, 182, 198–99; transition and transcendence narratives in, 19–22, 193; use of term, 23–24, 201, 207 n. 28

world-making projects, 6–7, 21–22, 24, 34, 59

Worsley, Jack, 210–11 n. 10

Wu Lien-The, 159, 227 n. 1

Xilu.com, 87, 101

xin (heart), 74, 79, 88

Xu Qing, 182–83

yajiankang (subhealth), 35, 45, 53–58, 66, 93

Yanagisako, Sylvia, 152, 154, 155, 213 n. 6

yi'an (medical cases) documentation, 107, 212 n. 4, 212 n. 5

yide (virtue of medical practice), 65–66, 84, 111

yisheng (doctor), 47, 203 n. 1

yishu (skill of medical practice), 65–66, 111

yuanmeng (fulfill a dream), and commodification, 86

Yueyang Hospital, 53, 68, 82, 204

yu shijie jiegui (get on track with the world) concept, 25, 34, 43–44, 61, 105, 176

zanfu systems, 76–77, 210 n. 9, 210–11 n. 10

Zhao Zhenjing, 92, 110

zhenjiuke, 212 n. 1. See also acupuncture

zhongchengyao (Chinese formula medicine), 18, 49, 113, 207 n. 23

Zhongguo Yishi Bowuguan (Museum of the History of Chinese Medicine), 145–47, 172

zhongyi (Chinese medicine), 5. See also traditional Chinese medicine

zhongyi waike (external medicine of traditional Chinese medicine), 83–84

Zhu Nanshan, 107–8, 109, 213 n. 7

Zhu Nansun, 213 n. 7

zuotang (sitting in the drugstore), and commodification, 82–83, 211 n. 17

MEI ZHAN is an associate professor
of anthropology at the University of
California, Irvine.

Library of Congress Cataloging-in-Publication Data
Zhan, Mei
Other-worldly: making Chinese medicine through
transnational frames / Mei Zhan
p. cm.
Includes bibliographical references and index.
ISBN 978-0-8223-4363-9 (cloth : alk. paper)
ISBN 978-0-8223-4384-4 (pbk. : alk. paper)
1. Medicine, Chinese. 2. Alternative medicine.
3. Integrative medicine. I. Title
R601.Z465 2009
616´09—dc22 2009022400